One-Handed
in a
Two-Handed
World *2nd Edition revised*

Prince Gallison Press books are available at special purpose quantity bulk purchase discounts, for sales promotions, premiums, fund-raising or educational use. Special books and or Book excerpts, can also be created to fit specific needs.

For details write or telephone the office of the Director of Special Markets, Prince Gallison Press
P.O. Box 23--Hanover Station
Boston, MA 02113
617-367-5815

One-Handed in a Two-Handed World

2nd Edition revised

- Tommye-Karen Mayer

Prince-
Gallison
Press

Boston, Massachusetts, 02113

One-Handed in a Two-Handed World, 2nd edition

Prince-Gallison Press, 2000, Revised August 2001

All Rights Reserved.

Copyright 2000 by Tommye-K. Mayer, Revised August 2001

Cover illustration copyright © 2000 by Prince-Gallison Press Revised 2001

Interior design by Tommye-K. Mayer

For information:

Prince-Gallison Press
P.O. Box 23, Hanover Station
Boston, MA 02113-0001
(tel) 617-367-5815
(fax) 617-367-3337
e-mail: princeg@gis.net

Library of Congress Catalog Card Number 99-90859

ISBN 0-9652805-1-9

Published in the United States
PRINTED IN THE UNITED STATES OF AMERICA
BFS Printers, Boston, MA

TABLE OF CONTENTS

FOREWORD

On my way home from work in June 1981, a blood vessel in my head burst. I've been *one handed in a two-handed world* ever since.

I was twenty-three years old when a half cup of blood flooded the right hemisphere of my brain. I'm told, it was such a serious bleed, few were convinced I'd survive. So I guess things were touch and go for a while that afternoon.

When I did survive, awakening from a coma a few days later, it was to a half-paralyzed body.

The *one-handedness part* of my hemi-paresis wasn't totally new to my family. My mother's father, we called him *Duke*, had learned to manage single-handedly after an industrial accident amputated his left wrist and hand long before I was born.

No one in the family mentioned Duke's hand, or discussed the accident. None of us did—not his four children or spouses, his nieces and nephews, his fifteen grandchildren their spouses, or his great grandchildren.

The accident had happened, that was all there was to it. We accepted the stump just as we accepted his adaptive techniques. That was the way he and my grandmother wanted it.

Duke never apologized for his missing left hand. He never even acknowledged its absence. We all witnessed his carrying on and succeeding despite it.

Mom speaks of the many times, when as a child and young girl, she'd *"hold the nail,"* while Duke swung the hammer. She never questioned. And he never missed.

Lot's of us manage single-handedly, and there are almost as many ways we get that way. For example every year:

☞ 39,000 are born one-handed or one-armed, or lose a hand or arm in accidents each year.[1]

☞ 3 million Americans survive stroke many living on with hemi-paresis.[2]

☞ Conservatively estimating, 14,000 Traumatically Brain Injured survive to live on without the use of one hand. [1]

☞ Some 350,000 Americans are missing a left or right arm or right hand. [1]

☞ Another 450,000 Americans live with a paralyzed left or right arm or hand. [1]

☞ As many as 4.5 million people suffer *Repetitive Strain injury*

them to manage single handedly for a period of time. [1]

☞ Countless *sporting injuries (from tennis elbow to breaks)* require people to manage single handedly both temporarily and permanently.

☞ Everyday accidents, while going about our daily business and at home cause long- and short-term one-handedness.

☞ Moms and dads with children not yet walking find themselves needing to manage with one hand as they continue on with activities of daily living while carrying a child perched on one hip. Embarrassed, new-parent-friends have asked, "how do I...?"

[1] Statistics from the 1992 National Health Interview Study.

[2] Statistic from the National Stroke Association

We one-handers have plenty of company. Whether you find yourself one-handed temporarily or permanently, this book is for you.

Why struggle through the several months your arm or hand is healing from a break, a strain, a sprain, burn, laceration, or surgery? Why reinvent the wheel for managing single-handedly?

If the doctor prescribed immobilization for your damaged arm or hand, or you've permanently lost use of an arm or hand, this book will help you get past the loss. Not only that, the tools identified here help you get back to participating in, and enjoying life despite it all.

After the hemorrhage, I wondered if I'd ever live independently again. Before the hemorrhage, that year after college, I'd left my hometown struggling to establish myself in Manhattan.

The hemorrhage and subsequent hemi-paralysis brought me to an acute-care hospital, a re-

habilitation hospital, and back to my parents home. While my folks truly have a lovely home, it is *their* home.

Now, two decades later and still single-handed, I don't live with my parents. I don't even live in the same town, though I do visit.

Thanks to my *Three Secrets* (*see page 11*), and the ways I've learned to apply them. I manage all my Activities of Daily Living (*ADLs*) single-handedly, and live independently, in the heart of downtown Boston.

While many of the ideas in the pages following might be easier if tried with help available—in case you get stuck—each is based on experience and has been accomplished alone.

* * * * *

I consider this book not so much as a set of skills as a methodology with examples to show you how to put that methodology into effect.

In this book, I share with you a system which I've found helpful in managing with one hand. My system resulted from a vivid dream I had while living at the rehabilitation hospital. The dream, and it's images remain with me today.

For the first time I saw my half-paralyzed self in a dream which had me stranded alone on a deserted island. It was as if the island's inhabitants had just evacuated, leaving my deserted island with all the *comforts & complexities* of home—even electricity.

The problem: I was alone on this island and I was one handed. Instead of being an intriguing and enticing fantasy, it became a nightmare.

How could I?... I was living in the rehabilitation hospital and hadn't tried cooking, or bathing myself—let alone washing and repairing clothes, or managing outdoors.

At the time of the dream, I felt utterly helpless, barely even dressing independently.

I awoke terrified, feeling useless, vulnerable, inadequate and hopeless. What this dream showed me was how much I needed to know I could do whatever I needed, for myself, by myself, and *hopefully* without too many special gadgets. Gadgets I might not have if ever I *were* on a deserted island.

So that's what this book is all about— learning to manage with one hand as though there's no one to take care of those allegedly *two-handed operations.*

Many benefits come from managing for yourself single-handedly. It isn't only reassuring, it also opens up new (*as well as reopens old*) options in life, and enables self-sufficiency.

Self-sufficiency and options beget healthy self-esteem, self-reliance, a more positive and optimistic outlook on life, greater self-assurance.

When first you lose, or lose the use of, a hand or arm, it's hard to look past everything, past all the many options that no longer seem open. This book helps you discover the many options still open, even those that seemed impossible.

It all seemed impossible to me too, though I've been fiercely independent since birth— always determined to be _grown up_. Grown-up, I defined as one-and-the-same-as _self-sufficient_.

Initially in my insistence at doing for myself, I too substituted by using my teeth and mouth for my lost _other_ hand. I quickly found relying on other people to do the simple tasks; putting toothpaste on the brush, shoe tying, opening cans,

selecting food at a buffet, depressing the public washroom faucet while I washed my hand, opening a soda can, and all those other tasks of everyday living, _drove me nuts,_ damaging what little self-esteem I had left.

It didn't take long to see I needed to know I could manage for myself with one hand. In striving for that goal, I've made myself figure out how to do _everything_ I need to do, for myself, by myself—_at least once._

My rule of thumb is to try something a few times. If, after trying, I find the effort involved in accomplishing _whatever_ is greater than the thrill of succeeding, next time, now that I know I _could_ manage in a pinch, I'm free to choose not to, and to ask for help.

Struggling with, and finally succeeding at, the hard stuff, makes it easier to ask for help. After trying and accomplishing, you can decide the effort is too much. That decision frees you to *choose* not to do it again, especially when a two-handed someone is more than willing to help.

Managing something difficult once, proves you can. Knowing you can, but mindfully asking for help, empowers.

Bottom line here, is by knowing the *Three Secrets* (*see next*), and making these secrets second nature, you' become confident you can manage anything that needs to be done for yourself.

That *knowing* helps rebuild the self-esteem that is so badly damaged when you lose the use of a hand, empowering you. The *knowing*, the self-esteem, and the empowerment are really the whole point of this book.

So, would I be able to manage on that island today? You bet.

And so will you once you internalize the *Three*

Secrets to managing single-handedly.

Good luck! And have fun with it. Everything you learn to do for yourself single-handedly is an accomplishment. You're not only *allowed* to pat yourself on the back with each breakthrough, you are *encouraged*.

I do!

THE THREE SECRETS

the core tenants to managing single-handedly, I call *The Three Secrets*. Always with you, are the two most critical tools for successfully negotiating this two-handed world single-handedly.

To successfully function with one hand, you need to learn how to use these *Three Secrets*, learn a few tricks of the trade, and pick up those mandatory gadgets.

1) Body Positioning

The First Secret to managing with one hand is "**Body Positioning**," understanding how you can organize yourself, enabling you to accomplish what you want. Sometimes you'll find all you need to do is figure out how to *position the limbs you can use* so your one hand can accomplish the project you've undertaken.

Learning to use your body to your best advantage includes deciding how and where to stand, for example, moving your torso to the left or right, or perhaps closer to your work station.

In the long run, "*Body Positioning*" is more important than finding tools to help accomplish tasks most people manage with two hands. You always have your body with you—there's no possibility of "*leaving it at home*" like that tool you have here somewhere...

Throughout this book, you'll see how to use *Body Position* in everyday life. Examples follow to help you see how to use the rest of you—_all_ the parts you have that still function—to accomplish what you want.

For example, perhaps by standing closer to the task at hand, you can use your abdomen to help leverage your project, keeping it from shifting position while you work on it. Throughout, you'll see suggestions relating to body position. After a while and with practice, facilitating activities with effective *Body Positioning* will become natural.

2) *Four Fingers and a Thumb*

The Second Secret to managing single-handedly is recognizing <u>you do not have *just one hand*</u>. Look again. You have *Four Fingers and a Thumb*.

Each of these digits works independently of the others. You can use your index finger separately from your thumb, and separately from your ring, your middle and your pinkie fingers, etc.

Think of it this way: Hands don't type, hands don't manipulate surgical instruments, hands don't play the guitar, the piano. *Fingers do.*

Those with the luxury of two hands often waste-

fully forego efficiently using each finger.

When you apply the consciousness of a classical guitarist to allocating the resources of your hand, all five resources— *all four fingers & thumb*— you can accomplish most of what you try. The rest gets finished up with the help of the First Secret, *"Body Positioning,"* and with the Third Secret.

You'll realize more of your goals once you learn to plan how you can best use your body to help you accomplish what you want, and truly understand *it isn't one hand. It's four fingers and a thumb.*

3) *Gadgets*

The Third Secret to man-aging single-handedly is **"Gadgets."** (*known by therapists as* A*SSISTIVE* D*EVICES*)

When *one-handedness* first happened to you, you may have thought the *Third Secret* was most important. N*ot so*. While a gadget can be key to accomplishing a specific task, gadgets can also be limiting.

It's great as long as you have the gadget you need when you need it. But when you don't? Especially if you travel, you may want to focus on adaptations enabling you to manage using *Four Fingers & a Thumb*, and *Body Positioning*.

That said, some gadgets are indispensable when managing with one hand: a *Cutting Board* (*see page 120*), a *Suction Cup Pad* (*see page 126*), a *Handled Sponge* (*see page 15)* and tools enabling you to participate in favorite leisure activities.

* * * * *

In that your experience and situation will inevitably be different from mine, or because you may be more enamored of gadgets than am I—they make terrific gifts, to give to yourself,

or to receive—I have looked at situations and described resolving each using *all three secrets*. If *Four Fingers and a Thumb* or *Body Positioning* don't work for you, by all means try a gadget—one I've described, or something you discover for yourself.

Throughout this book the solutions relying on *body positioning, four fingers and a thumb, or gadgets* give you examples for manipulating what you have such that doing it can even resemble *sleight of hand* to the uninitiated. I hope you have a lot of fun with these tips and with the freedom and independence you regain once you've learned to manage *One-Handed in this Two-Handed World*.

PERSONAL CARE

Let's focus on the basics to start—things they took care of for you while you were in the hospital, or that immediately after the onset of single-handedness family and friends do for you. People will wash your hair for you, give you sponge baths, and prepare your tooth brush—for a while. In the beginning, they'll even bend over and tie your shoes for you.

Inevitably, despite good intentions, they scrub too vigorously or not vigorously enough, the water isn't the right temperature, too warm or too cool. They don't wash everywhere. There's still a film of soap on your hair after the final rinse. There's too much or too little toothpaste. Or your feet don't feel right in your shoes—too loose or cramped.

Complaining seems ungrateful. But then again, why shouldn't you yearn for the creature comforts grown-up two-handed people enjoy? The best way to get something done the way you like it, is managing it for yourself.

Bathing

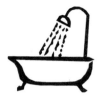

Despite one-handedness, bathing is essential—*cleanliness is next to godliness.* Not only will you look and smell good, once you can do it for yourself again, you'll feel better. It all seems to improve when you look and smell pleasant, with clean hair too. Not only that, the rest of the world seems more welcoming. Despite your disability (*be it temporary or permanent*), you need to practice good hygiene. Just see how doable it is, even one handedly.

Grab bars

Losing the use of a hand or arm can dramatically affect your sense of balance. Grab bars—steel handrails designed for the bathroom—come in many different lengths and can be installed in most bathrooms and showers with a minimum of fuss, especially now in these post-ADA (*Americans with Disabilities Act*) days. More carpenters or handymen/women have experience installing Grab Bars.

Consider having a Grab Bar added to your shower or bath area, even if your injury is temporary. As you age, balance tends to change. Who knows, you might need a grab bar again later on. *For information on how to obtain a* **Grab Bar** *turn to* **Resources***, beginning page 246.*

Handled Sponges

Maybe you've already discovered that washing the armpit under the arm you use isn't easy. Your one hand *just doesn't bend that way.* You can resolve this problem with a bottle sponge. You'll find one wherever you buy dish washing liquid and your other sponges. Or try a **Handled Sponge** (*pictured left*).

To wash the armpit under the arm you use, grab your Handled sponge by the handle. Wet the sponge and rub it over your bar of soap (*you can leave the soap in the soap dish to do this—no need to pick up the soap bar*). Now just rub the soaped sponge under your arm. To rinse, wet the sponge and swipe the now water-laden sponge under your arm. *For information obtaining a Handled Sponge see* **Resources,** *beginning page 246.*

Shower Brush

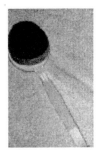

While most of what you do in the shower or bath only requires one hand, or one hand at a time, you'll find *a Shower Brush* indispensable for back, leg—just about all-over—washing.

Once you're inside the shower, the easiest way to get soap on your shower brush is to rub the soap bar against the small of your back with your one hand.

After you've raised lather, rinse your one hand, and pick up the back brush (*You'll find it easier if you use a back brush that can be hung in an accessible place inside your shower*) now with a massaging circular stroke, rub the bristles of the shower brush in the lather at the small of your back. Enlarge the circle until you've soaped your whole back. Turn around, and while you're rinsing off your back, you can soap up your front side, scrub legs and haunches, then rinse front.

Drying off

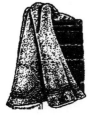

You've probably already found toweling dry the regular way, with a bath towel, isn't satisfactory. Getting your back dry is really a two-handed operation. If you were accustomed to bringing your clothes into the bathroom with you, quickly toweling dry, and emerging fully dressed, ready for the day, you've probably been disappointed. Toweling dry single-handedly just doesn't easily dry your back.

* * * * *

You may even have tried holding one corner of the towel, tossing the rest of the towel over your shoulder and dragging it across your back, one shoulder at a time, probably only to discover it's _okay_, but it only takes care of the wetness and your skin is still damp. Even after two or three passes on each side!

It's hard to feel clean and comfortable when your clothes stick to a damp mist all over your body. You've probably said to yourself, _there has to be another way._

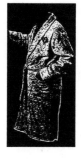

Well there is!

* * * * *

Cotton Terrycloth Bathrobe. Not only are terrycloth robes warm and cozy to curl up on the sofa, with a good book. If you put on your terrycloth robe as you step out of the shower, it'll thoroughly dry off not just your back, but most of your body too—except your hair, hand(s), lower legs, and feet. Don't toss out the towels... but *do* get a terrycloth robe!

Eyes / Contact Lenses

You can insert, remove, and clean contact lenses using four fingers and a thumb. My first experience with glasses and contacts was after I lost use of my hand.

Here are my suggestions:

Inserting the lens

If your Optometrist approves, use one of the new *Multi-Purpose Contact Lens Solutions*. These solutions are used to clean, rise, disinfect, and store your contact lenses.

To manage lenses single-handedly, you need to set aside a table at which you can sit and use only for your contacts. On this table lay a wash cloth as if it were a place mat and across from the chair set up a make-up mirror. (*The best mirror choice managing contacts single-handedly is a lighted magnification mirror.*) Also on this table should be the cleaning solution and your lens case—everything you need for your contacts.

Before sitting down to insert or remove your contact lenses, always wash your one hand (*your fingers get into a lot of places and your eyes shouldn't be the last place they go since you washed them...*)

Now you're ready to insert your lenses. With the lens case resting on the wash cloth on your table, unscrew the cover of one lens cup by holding the lens case pressed against the length of your thumb with the cover of the cup you to be opened between your thumb pad and the side of your index finger pad, and the other lens cup leveraged against the heel of your hand and tip of your ring finger.

Twist the cap between your thumb and index finger to loosen it. As the cap loosens, you can relax your hold on the lens case, friction of the case on the wash cloth should provide enough resistance.

When the cover is free of the threads, lift it off and place it down on your wash cloth. Dip your index finger into the lens cup, fitting the tip of your finger into the curve of the contact lens and draw the lens up the side of the cup and out on your index fingertip.

Clean your lens by gently rubbing it with your thumb pad. After a few rubs (*when it stops feeling "oily"*) Pick the lens off your index finger pad, with your thumbnail, onto the wash cloth rounded side up, this way "⌒". Drip a few drops of lens solution on the lens, then lightly touch the curve of the lens with the tip of your index finger, if the lens doesn't stick to the tip of your index finger drip another drop of solution over the lens, being careful not to drip so much that you flatten the lens, turning it in-side-out. (*If it does turn in-side-out, not to worry. Drip another drop of lens solution into the lens and with the tips of your thumb and index finger pads press down on the edge of the lens, turning it right-side-up and looking like this "⌒" again.*)

Once again, lightly touch the curve of the lens with the tip of your index finger. Keep trying until the lens sticks to the tip of your finger alternating between dampening your index fingertip and the rounded, convex surface of the lens. *The first time you try putting in your contacts it may take a number of tries. With practice it does get easier.*

With the lens concave on your index fingertip, like this "⌣" lift your finger up toward your eye. Raise your eyebrow to open your upper eyelid and with the tip of your middle fingertip gently pull down the lower eyelid.

Lightly touch the lens to your eyeball. Your upper lid will reflexively want to close. Fight that reflex. Instead gently roll your eyeball and with your index and ring fingers resting on your cheekbone and your middle finger on your lower lid, ease your lower lid up and over your pupil, seating the contact lens.

This is one place where the mirror comes in handy,

enabling you to verify that the lens is properly placed on your pupil and not hung up on your eyelashes.

One down, one to go... Replace the cover on the lens cup that you just finished using, and repeat these steps for your other eye.

With practice, and fairly quickly, this process does get easier, so that fairly shortly you can manipulate your contacts when you're away from home. But be sure to set up a space away from home bounded by a wash cloth. Two-handed people use the palm of their "*other hand*" as their workspace when cleaning and manipulating their lenses. Single-handedly, we use readily available wash cloths on a table surface.

Removing the lens

Open your eye wide. With your middle finger draw down the lower eyelid for the eye holding the contact lens you're taking out. With the tip of your index finger pad and the tip of your thumb pad lightly touching your eyeball straddling the pupil just outside the lens, _gently pinch your thumb and middle finger together_, picking the lens off your eyeball.

With the lens gently pinched between your thumb and middle finger, place it concave, like this "U" on your wash cloth. Drip a couple drops of *Multi-Purpose Contact Solution* into the lens. Touch the your index finger pad into the lens. The lens will stick to your fingertip allowing you to pick up the lens. Turn your hand palm and index finger pad up. Gently rub the lens between your index finger and thumb, cleaning the lens. When the lens no longer feels "*oily*" peel the lens off your index finger pad with the edge of your thumbnail and back onto the wash cloth. Drip a few more drops of *Multi-Purpose Contact Solution* into the lens to rinse off the proteins dislodged from the lens by your rubbing. You are now ready to return this lens to its cup in your lens case.

One down, one to go... Repeat this process with your other eye's lens. *Again, with practice, this part of managing contact lenses single-handedly gets easier too.*

Hair

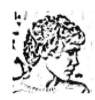

Your hair is one of the first things people notice about you. Spending time learning manage it single-handedly, so it looks as attractive as possible, will help you realize your personal, professional, and social goals.

If you don't *look* capable, people assume you aren't, and won't explore further. Your hair needs to be clean, and well groomed for every day and for going out, no matter how hard that **seems** now.

Washing

Some people—one-handed and two-handed—deal with hair washing and styling by fitting three or more hairdresser appointments a week into the schedule and budget. If a solution like this works with your temperament, your lifestyle, and budget, why not? But if you want or need to take care of hair washing and styling for yourself single-handedly, you can.

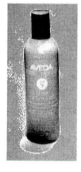

Flip-top bottles and tubes are the simplest containers to use single-handedly. Not only is the cap attached to the bottle while you apply the shampoo, but the amount you squeeze out is controlled by the smaller "*pin hole*" opening.

Before stepping into the shower, on days you plan to wash your hair, clean the hair out of your hairbrush, and bring your hairbrush into the shower with you.

Now you're ready. Position your head under the water flow. Completely wet your hair. With your one hand slick your wet hair back, off your forehead.

Pick up the shampoo bottle and tip your head back, away from the water, so you're almost looking up at the ceiling.

To make it easier to check the amount of shampoo you use, point the shampoo bottle spout at your forehead just below your hairline, squeeze as you draw the bottle along your hairline, leaving a thin line of shampoo along the top of your forehead just below your hairline.

By doing it this way, you can feel, against your forehead skin just how much shampoo you're using. Stop when it feels like you've got enough shampoo to work up a good lather, and put down the bottle.

With your one hand massage the shampoo throughout and into your hair, working up the beginning of a good lather. Now rinse off your one hand and pick up your hair brush.

With your hairbrush, scrub your hair, massaging your scalp. Using your hair brush this way is almost the same as giving yourself a _salon-like_ scalp massage, and it helps to work up a rich thick lather. Not only will your hair be squeaky clean and your scalp tingling, but your hair brush will be as clean as your hair and you won't be brushing the oils that had collected on the bristles when you last brushed your hair, back into your freshly washed, shiny clean hair.

Styling

As important as keeping your hair clean, is making sure that the style you've chosen is: **1)** Appropriate for your hair type, **2)** Appropriate to your looks, **3)** Appropriate to your lifestyle, and **4)** Appropriate to your single-handedness.

Get the Best Cut

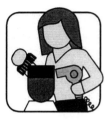

First, find a hairdresser who sees her/himself as a professional, someone to whom you can say, "*This is the face. This is the hair. I can't and won't do complicated styling. What do you recommend for me?*"

If the hairdresser hands you a magazine and asks you to find something you like, go somewhere else. A professional will be able to tell you by looking at your face and by examining the type of hair you have, what cut will work best for you. A professional takes into consideration the size and shape of your face, the weight and thickness of your hair, your lifestyle and physical limitations. S/he will then describe the cut.

Go with it.

This is the surest way to realize the ultimate *wash and wear hair* cut. Don't worry. If you really hate the cut—most likely that won't be the case 'cause you'll love it—in just a few months your hair will grow back, and you can try something else with someone else.

Women

So now that you've got *wash and wear hair*, what can you do to spruce it up for special occasions? To give yourself a change, you **can** single-handedly manage curlers, gels, and mousse.

Rollers

Just because the rollers you once used aren't *one-handable*, doesn't mean you're out of luck. You can still curl your hair.

All you need are the *right* ones. Velcro, the wonder product compliments of our NASA space program, makes the single-handed roller a reality. Your hair *sticks* to the **Velcro roller**, and the rollers *stick* to each other as you put in the next one, so there's no need for an *other hand*. Wonder why anyone uses any other kind of roller. *For information on how to obtain Velcro Rollers see* **Resources**, *page* 246.

Mousse

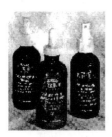

The way to work with Mousse is to squirt your "*lemon sized mound*" onto the porcelain flat edge around your bathroom sink. (*If there isn't a flat edge, try squirting the mound right into the dry sink bowl.*) After you've put down the mousse can, mush about half of that mound into the palm of your one hand. Now comb your fingers through the hair on one half of your head, wiping the palm of your hand against your hair. It'll take a few passes to work the Mousse through your hair. Now scoop the rest of the Mouse into your hand and comb your fingers, wiping your palm, through the other half of your hair.

Gel

Because it's more *liquidy*, you'll handle gel differently from mousse.

*   *   *   *   *

New!

Working over a sink or table, flip open the Gel container top. Straddling the *pinhole* opening with the palm of your hand, your thumb pressing against the side of the squeeze bottle, your index, middle, and ring fingers pressing against the opposite side. Tip the squeeze bottle up-side-down so the *pinhole* opening points down into the palm of your hand. Hold the bottle that way for a moment or two, allowing gravity to move the Gel inside toward the *pinhole* opening. Now squeeze your thumb and fingers together. Stop squeezing when you have a quarter-sized mound in your palm. Lower your hand toward the sink or table, releasing your thumb's pressure on the bottle and balancing the squeeze bottle on your fingers. You don't want to turn your hand palm-side-down lest the Gel plop to the sink/table. Not to worry, gravity, finger positioning and working with the sink/table enable you to lower the Gel squeeze bottle to the sink/table in a position such that the contents won't leak out while you work the gel through your hair.

Once you've stashed the gel bottle, work your fingers around your palm coating your palm, fingers, and thumb with Gel. Now comb your fingers through your hair—both sides of your head. ☺ Don't forget... your one hand is responsible for combing through *all* your hair with Gel. If you run out on one side, squeeze some more gel into the palm of your hand, mush it around again—you don't want a blob of Gel in any one place...

Now with the Gel in your hair, style as you like and or blow dry (*see page 29 for ideas on hair drying*).

* * * * *

Alternatively try laying your comb on the flat edge around your bathroom sink, or in the dry sink bowl if there is no flat edge. Squeeze a thin stripe of gel across the comb teeth about half-way down the teeth, the full length of the comb. Pick up the comb, being careful to keep it as flat as you can, and comb half the length of it through the hair on one half of your head. You may find it easier to start working with the same side as the arm you use.

Then run the half of the comb still striped with the Gel through the other side of your hair. After a few passes through your hair with the comb, put down the comb. For more body and shape, touch up the gel application by picking at and mussing your hair with your fingertips.

Men

You, too, must be sure to get yourself the best cut—Men's hairstyles have come a long way since numbered barbershop cuts. You too can have _wash and wear_ hair. Consult with a hair stylist—for details on this, _turn to page 25._

Once you've gotten that easy-to-manage cut, you can also try Mousse or Gel, (_see page 26_)—It's the dawn of the twenty-first century, guys. That _greasy kid stuff_ look is out. Besides, new hair-styling products make managing hair single-handedly almost easy.

Hair Drying

It is nice to be able to maybe tease your hair a bit, with your fingers, a comb, or brush while the hair dryer blows—rather difficult if your one hand is occupied holding the hair dryer. There is a solution: a wall mounted _Hair Dryer Holder_ (pictured left) mounted on the wall with three suction cups, or with screws. _For information on obtaining your **Hair Dryer Holder** see_ **Resources**_, page 246._

Nail Care

Maintaining the fingernails on the hand you use is critical. Not only is the condition of the nails on this hand you use highly noticeable, but use makes your nails on that one hand more subject to chips, tears, and breakage. Besides, short, well-kept fingernails are useful tools when managing single-handedly.

You may have enjoyed long fingernails before you temporarily or permanently lost the use of your *other hand*, but you'll find that long nails just don't work when you're single-handed.

Emery Boards

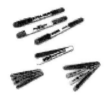

Because emery boards are rough on both sides, by laying an emery board on your trouser-clad thigh (the leg on the same side as the arm you use), you can file the fingernails on the hand you use by stroking each nail along the length of the emery board resting on your thigh, the "*other*" side of the emery board will "*stick*" to your trousers. If you're diligent, and don't let your fingernails grow too long, you may be able to take care of your fingernails this way, using only an emery board—at least until you get your own *Nail Care System,* that is. (*See next.*)

Nail Care System

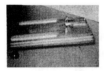

For nails that grow too quickly or thick to be maintained with an emery board alone, or when you tire of filing, try a *Nail Care System.* This clever product consists of an attractively finished wooden platform with suction cup feet to hold it in place at one end and a large nail clipper attached to the platform so its lever-handle protrudes through a hole. The platform is also fitted with cutouts to hold two standard nail files—making both the finer polishing surface and the coarser surface readily accessible.

To use the *Nail Care System*, set it on a table at a comfortable height and rest your hand on the board with your fingers outstretched. Slide the fingernail you want to clip between the upper and lower nail clipper cutting edges. Press down on the board. This forces the lever-handle of the nail clipper against the table closing the cutting edges to over your fingernail, clipping it just where you wanted. With practice you'll soon perfect the process. *See* **Resources**, *page 246 for information on obtaining a Nail Care System.*

Skin Care

Skin care isn't just your hand and face. While those are the first skin other people notice, for your personal comfort and well-being, you need to take care of *all* your skin single-handedly, even that "*hard-to-reach*" skin.

Back Itch

When the itch is just beyond your reach, you can try explaining to someone just exactly where it itches and how much. Somehow though, that never seems terribly effective. After all the: "*Over, over,*" "*Up there,*" "*No, no, over there,*" "*Too, too much,*" "*Up, up,*" "*There, there,*" "*No, there,*" it's hardly worth the effort, especially when half the time it *still* itches afterward.

* * * * *

Back scratchers work, assuming you near by when the need arises. back scratchers make *great* gifts for single-handers.

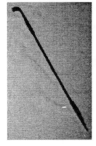

* * * * *

For those times when you're in urgent need, no one's around, and your back scratcher is no where to be found, try this:

Stand in an inside doorway with your feet about shoulder width apart straddling the threshold. Roll your shoulders forward so your back is rounded. Swaying side to side, rub your back against the door jamb. The uneven planes will help you get that itch yourself, quickly and effectively.

It won't be long before two-handed friends do the same when the unreachable itch strikes. I've seen mine straddling threshold, swaying in the doorway.

One way to keep down the number of itches, back and otherwise, is to take care your skin is clean and moisturized.

Moisturizer

Many bar soaps moisturize while cleaning, so as you lather, you're also moisturizing.

Alternatively use a large rubber spatula to spread skin lotion on your back. Exactly how to do this is described in *"Sun Screen,"* the next section.

Sun screen

Even the two-handed find applying suntan lotion to their own backs problematic. The bottom line here is, there's no shame in asking someone to rub suntan lotion on your back, everyone else does.

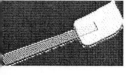

However, if your back will be exposed to the sun, you can protect yourself with suntan lotion for yourself by using a large *rubber spatula*. Lean forward (*it helps ensure the lotion doesn't dribble*) and squirt a half-dollar sized puddle of lotion on the small of your back. Put down the lotion bottle, and pick up the spatula.

Using the same stroke you'd use to frost a cake with a spatula, push the lotion around the lower part of your back. When you've finished spreading lotion over this first section, straighten up, and put down the spatula. Pick up the lotion bottle again. Lean over and squirt another half-dollar sized puddle of lotion, now in the center of your back, about halfway up.

Pick up the spatula. Reaching behind you spread the lotion on your back. When you're done with the middle third of your back, sit up and put down the spatula.

When you're ready to finish up, lean over again, pick up the lotion and squirt another half-dollar sized puddle of lotion, high up on your back, just below your neck, between your shoulders. Pick up the spatula and spread the lotion over this last third of your back. You're done with your back now, but you're still not quite ready to get dressed.

It's especially important not to forget to protect the arm you use with suntan lotion, and particularly that shoulder. In order to take care of the arm you use, put the lotion on while you're still only wearing your undies unless you're getting into a swimsuit or shorts. To put lotion on the arm and shoulder of the hand you use, the leg on the same side as the hand you use needs to be uncovered.

Sit on the edge of a chair with your feet shoulder-width apart, soles flat on the floor. Squeeze a half-dollar size puddle of sun lotion on the _outside_ of the knee on the side as the hand you use.

Raise the knee with the lotion on it by pressing your toes into the floor so you lift your heel off the ground. Lean forward, extending the hand you use toward the floor, with your elbow straight. Dab the inside point of your shoulder into the puddle of lotion.

With the inside point of your shoulder touching the puddle of lotion, begin straightening to a sitting position. As you straighten upright, drag and rotate your arm through the puddle of lotion. Lower your heel to the floor to help spread the lotion down to your wrist and over the fingers you use. Lean forward and straighten again a few times more to rub the lotion into the skin.

When that first puddle of lotion is *used up* and spread on the arm you use, squeeze a second half-dollar sized puddle on the *inside* of the same knee, the knee on the same side as the hand you use. Lean forward again, with your elbow straight and now press the highest outside part of your shoulder into the middle of the puddle. Pull up, to your upright sitting position, dragging and rotating your arm through the lotion puddle, and rubbing it into your skin. Repeat as necessary.

Shaving

Men

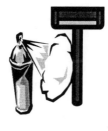

If your one hand is your dominant hand, you probably won't have much difficulty learning to shave single-handedly. But if your one hand is the nondominant, this may be the time to try an electric shaver. When shopping, take extra time in selecting your electric shaver, making sure it comfortably fits your one hand, and checking you can easily disassemble it for cleaning, and routine maintenance.

Women

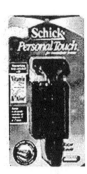

If your one hand is your dominant hand, shaving your legs using one hand probably won't be so much of a problem. Though you may find getting to the back and far side of the leg opposite the hand you use feels awkward. With practice, you'll get used to it.

Shaving under the one arm you use can be problematic, especially if the hand you use isn't your dominant one. The thicker and longer, curved handled women's razors are easier to manage single-handedly because of that curved handle, and the added length. By holding the razor close to the end of its handle, you can reach the blade to shave under your arm. Women's razors also tend to be lighter-weight which helps when holding so close to the end.

If a razor doesn't work for you, that's okay. Why not try a depilatory? Just wipe on a cream wait a few minutes and then rinse the hair off your legs. To apply the cream under your arm, use a sponge with a handle (*see page 15*). Consider owning two of these handled sponges—one for washing and the other for the depilatory— just in case all the depilatory doesn't rinse out last time you "*shave.*"

Teeth

Brushing

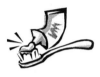

Select toothpaste tubes with _"flip-top"_ covers or _pump dispensers_. Flip-tops eliminate unscrewing tiny toothpaste caps, which inevitably fall to the floor rolling to an inaccessible somewhere.

Since squeezing the toothpaste tube or pump requires a hand, and holding the toothbrush to receive what you squeeze out requires another hand, single-handedly, you need to be creative.

At home, you can lay your toothbrush on the flat porcelain sink edge and squeeze paste onto the brush that way, but if you travel, consider some of these other ideas. All sorts of things go on in bathrooms and they're hard a to keep clean enough for resting something that you're about to put into your mouth!

* * * * *

Try clenching the toothbrush handle between your teeth so the bristles stand upright. With the toothpaste in your one hand, squeeze some onto those bristles. Once you've got the right amount on the brush, stash the toothpaste where ever it goes, and with your one hand remove the toothbrush handle from your mouth, take hold of it, normally, and brush.

One single-handed woman I know resolves her toothpaste/toothbrush problem by squirting paste directly into her mouth, stashing the paste, picking up her brush, and brushing.

* * * * *

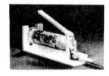

You can also try the ***Toothpaste Dispenser System***. Not only is the dispenser designed to squeeze out *just the right amount of toothpaste*, but it also holds your toothbrush in a slot with the bristles positioned to receive that *"just right amount"* exactly where you want it, evenly spread across the bristles. *For information on how to obtain a* **Toothpaste Dispenser System** *see* **Resources**, *beginning on page 246.*

* * * * *

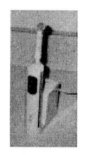

Electric toothbrushes, designed to massage your gums and remove plaque and tartar build-up are easily managed single-handedly. You can clip the toothbrush onto the motorized element/handle containing the rechargeable battery just once, leaving it set-up permanently. Or, by clenching the motorized element/handle between your thighs, you can pick up the toothbrush in your one hand and snap it into the motorized element/handle.

To apply toothpaste, lay the element/handle in the sink bowl. Pick up your toothpaste tube and squeeze the toothpaste onto the bristles of the brush.

Or, clenching the element/handle between your knees, apply the toothpaste.

Flossing

If you've seen your dentist since your one-handedness happened, your dental hygienist probably already admonished you for not flossing regularly. No doubt, toward the end of your appointment, she quickly and efficiently wrapped dental floss around each of her *two* index fingers and flossed around your every tooth.

You've probably already discovered that off-the-shelf dental floss is designed for two-handed use, and isn't manageable single-handedly. The dental floss handles, designed for those who don't care to stick their fingers inside their mouths, require an *other* hand to set-up.

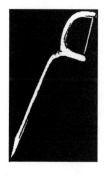

Single-handedly, you can floss using plastic *disposable* **Flossers**. These relatively inexpensive adaptations are small enough carry in your change purse or pocket, or to stash in the pencil organizer in your desk drawer, and have whenever needed. Or arrange them in a shot glass-sized container on a shelf in the bathroom. *For information on how to obtain* **Flossers** *see* **Resources**, *page 246.*

Bandaging

New!

With your one hand and arm as busy as they are managing single-handedly, it's inevitable that one or both will get *damaged*—cut, burnt, whatever, at some point. So there you are, with dirt and gunk in a bleeding wound, after falling, or maybe it's a kitchen, or working around the home cut or scrape injury. It needs to be cleaned and bandaged.

You *can* do this single-handedly.

Using whatever parts of your body you can; fingers, elbow, shoulder, knee, hip, etc., *get yourself inside and at a sink* with a clean washcloth, dishcloth, towel, some material. *Turn on the water* somehow, with which ever digits or limb, you have available (*I've done it with the bend of my elbow, a pinkie, my nose*) turn the water on warm. You need to clean this wound.

Hold the wound under the stream of water. This will wash off the larger bits of dirt and the blood, enabling you to take a look, assess the damage. It will also help clean out the bottom of the sink a bit. *Wet the cloth,* then *line the bottom of the sink with it, covering the cloth with water*. Now *draw the wound over the submerged cloth*—yes it'll hurt, but you have to clean this injury

Gently, and diligently *draw the wound across the cloth, cleaning it*, adding soap as appropriate. Regularly check the wound, you don't want to aggravate the injury by washing too vigorously, just enough to cleanse it.

When it's clean to your satisfaction, _lay a clean dry towel_ or cloth _on a counter_ or table and firmly but gently _press the injury into the cloth, blotting off the water_.

Now you're ready to bandage. Lay out on the counter what materials you have on hand—adhesive bandages, gauze, first aid tape, antibiotic salve. Before bandaging, you need to put salve on the injury. If you're wearing long pants but can bring the pant leg up over your knee, sit down. Otherwise, unbuckle your belt, drop your pants below you knees and sit down close enough to reach your first aid supplies.

Squeeze a dollop of salve on your knee on the same side as your wound—enough salve to thoroughly cover the injury. Wipe the injury across the dollop of salve, spreading the salve over the injury, but not too far into the surrounding skin where the salve would interfere with the adhesive bandage or tape's ability to stick.

Depending on the size of the wound and the bandages you have available, lay out the bandaging using what ever portion of your hand or body you can (pinky finger and thumb, mouth, elbow, ring finger, the heel of your hand, nose, toes...).

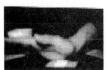

Photo by JoAnne N. Mayer

If you have adhesive bandages such as Band-Aids,® open the quantity you need to cover the wound. Lay out the bandages adhesive-side up side-by-side. Press the wound into the bandages, rocking to adhere the adhesive.

If it's gauze and first aid tape you're working with, while I don't like suggesting it, but most professional First-Aid folks do, use your teeth to rip the tape into usable lengths. Again, depending on the size of the wound, rip off three to five lengths of tape, lay these on the table adhesive side up, then lay the gauze on top of the tape, and press the wound into the gauze rolling your arm/hand over the adhesive tape to adhere it to your skin.

Done.

If it's a serious injury, it might be wise to have a medical someone take a look now that you're "*travelable*." Otherwise, after you wake up, you need to take a look at the injury, perhaps wash it again, put on more salve and re-bandage as necessary until you're healed.

I am so sorry you needed to refer to this section. Hope you're back in performance shape again soon.

DRESSING

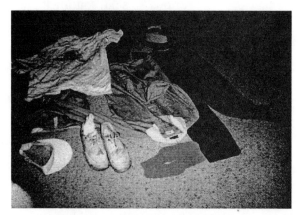

Some articles of clothing will be easier to manage single-handedly than others. For easy dressing, Snaps, buttons, and Velcro are best. Another invaluable feature for well-dressed one-handers is *Pockets*. Especially pockets located at your hip, on the same side as the hand you use.

Undergarments

Especially in colder climates, single-handed, men and women, need to work out managing their undergarments.

Women

Brassieres

Half-dressed, totally frustrated, and lying in bed in the rehabilitation hospital, I was in a state when a school friend I'd last seen at our fifth reunion, about a year ago walked in, visiting unexpectedly.

"How are you?" she asked.

"Furious!" I said, spitting it out.

I'd nearly turned myself inside out trying to take off the *one-size-fits-all* bra I'd so confidently pulled on that morning. Just the week before, I'd discovered I didn't know how to handle the front hook bras I'd worn before the hemorrhage.

"Why bother?" my friend asked, looking at me. "You don't *have* to wear a bra, you know."

I looked at braless her, and then down realizing she was probably right.

Improved!

> Now why I never thought about slipping the shoulder straps off my shoulders, sliding my arms out and then bringing the bra down past my waist, over my hips and then off at my feet, I'll never know. This method *does* work, though the bra does get rather twisted up.

You can straighten out the twists by putting your one hand through the shoulder straps and shaking the bra.

* * * * *

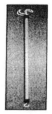

Alternatively, another trick to getting a bra off is having the right tool. Try using a **Dressing Stick** to reach over your shoulder and behind. Hook the back strap of your bra and pull the bra up to your shoulders and then over your head. *For information*

*on obtaining **Dressing Stick**, see **Resources**, page 246.*

Camisoles

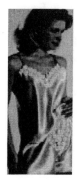

If after trying to deal with a bra single-handedly, you decide your figure really doesn't require you wear one, you may want to try a camisole. Camisoles made of lacy nylon or cotton, feel warm the winter. And in the summer, a finely woven cotton camisole helps absorb perspiration. Wearing camisoles might not be just an adaptation—it may actually become your preference.

Pantyhose

As long as properly dressed women must wear nylons, you do too. The trick for us, is in choosing the right pantyhose. We need nylons sturdy enough to pull on single-handedly without poking our four fingers and thumb through the weave as we pull.

After trying dozens of styles, I finally discovered ***L'eggs Sheer Energy*** can consistently be single-handedly drawn over foot, one at a time, pulled up over the shins, then quite aggressively grabbed with one hand, and fitted over thighs. *See* **Resources**, *page 246 for how to obtain **L'eggs Sheer Energy Pantyhose** inexpensively.*

Men

T-shirts

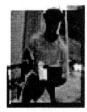

Lay your T-shirt flat on the bed, front down with the hem at the edge of the bed, closest to you. Lift the back of the T-shirt, at the midpoint of the bottom hem. With your one hand slide *the arm for the hand you don't use* into the T-shirt, guiding it into its armhole and sleeve.

Once the T-shirt shoulder is properly seated over the shoulder of the *arm for the hand you don't use*, slide the hand you use toward its arm opening, and through. Wiggle that shoulder into place. The T-shirt will be a band across your chest. Lift the back of the T-shirt by the hem, holding it in the center. Pull the back hem up and toward your head. Duck your head inside the shirt, through the neck opening.

Taking off your T-shirt single-handedly is easiest if you reach with your one hand behind your head, grab hold of your T-shirt close to the neck and pull it over your head from the back. If the front neck opening gets stuck on your chin—not to worry—let go of the back, and from the front ease your chin and nose through the hole, then reach back again and pull your T-shirt over your head.

After a while you'll get used to how your head needs to duck, perhaps pressing your chin against your chest or turning your head to one side, so your chin and nose don't get hung up on the neck hole as you pull off your T-shirt.

Boxer/Jockey Shorts

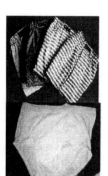

Sit down on the edge of your bed or on a chair, with the waistband of your boxer/jockey shorts across your lap, the fly/front on top. Take hold of the waistband of your boxer/jockey shorts by wrapping your one hand, palm to fingers around the front of the waistband.

Pick up your boxer/jockey shorts, and leaning forward, slide the back of the waistband and the seat of your shorts over your knees. Step into them with one leg. (*If the leg opposite your one hand isn't affected[1], it's quicker to start with that leg.*) That way, between your one hand and the opposite leg, you can hold the waistband open and easily slip your other leg in. Now, pull them up either by gently rocking side to side and pulling up, or stand up.

---

[1] If you're are not only one-handed, but also hemiplegic, as am I, it is *not* easier to start with your affected leg which would be the leg opposite the arm you use. Getting that leg in becomes a feat in and of itself... Instead, slip your unaffected leg in first. Move your hand across your chest, so that you're holding the waistband at the same side as your affected leg. Now you can maneuver the waistband forward and down, pulling the waistband taut between the hand you use and your unaffected leg. scoop the waistband under your affected foot, using the waistband to guide that foot in.

Tops

Women

It's easier to wear tops with generous sleeves, especially if you're wearing a cast or brace on that *other arm*. Even if you're not wearing a cast or brace, it's easier to feed your *other arm* into a sufficiently roomy shirt sleeve.

Pullovers, Turtlenecks, Sweaters

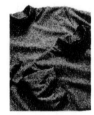

Start by laying out the turtleneck on the bed with the tag inside, but on top, That way when you pick up the turtleneck you'll put the back on your back and the front on your front.

Lift up the bottom opening and first feed the arm you don't use inside and into its sleeve. Follow by slipping the arm you use into its sleeve. Now, duck your head inside, and with the help of your one hand, slip your head through the neck hole. Wriggle the shoulder corresponding to the hand you use to settle the turtleneck shoulder onto you shoulders.

Pull down on the hem all around to seat it comfortably on both shoulders and around your neck.

Taking off your pullover turtleneck single-handedly, is easiest if you reach with your one hand behind your head, and grab hold of your turtleneck close to the neck and pull it over your head from the back.

If the front of the neck opening gets stuck on your chin, just let go of the back and from the front ease your chin and nose through, then reach back again and pull your sweater/turtleneck over your head.

Blouses

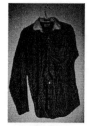

Most blouses fasten with buttons. You can manage buttons with the help of the following tips.

*   *   *   *   *

Pro baseball pitcher, Jim Abbott, who also happens to be one-handed, resolves the buttoning problem by leaving his game jersey in his locker already buttoned. Before game time, he slips it over his head like a pullover. This method only works with "*men-cut*" shirts. Women's "*blouses*," tapered at the waist, are often too narrow to pull overhead.

Cuff Buttons

If you can "*fold*" the-hand-you-use (*press your thumb against your pinkie finger*) tightly enough, and slide your hand through the sleeve and cuff with the cuff already buttoned, you've dealt with that cuff button. If you can't fold your hand narrow enough, try moving the cuff button on that sleeve closer to the edge of the cuff. (*for help with this turn to page 161,* **Hand Sewing**) If moving the button doesn't give you enough room to slip your hand through, re-sew the button with elastic thread. That should give you enough room to slide your hand through the cuff. Another trick is to choose blouses with elastic at the cuff.

Before you start buttoning your blouse up the front, line up the shirttails. There's absolutely nothing worse than single-handedly buttoning a bunch of buttons, only to find you've got an extra button-hole at the top, and a button at the bottom, Now you have to undo them all, and start all over again.

Overlay the line of buttons with the placket of buttonholes This is easiest to do in front of a mirror, but you *can* manage when a mirror isn't available, by matching the shirttails in front at the bottom corners and pulling down.

To button the buttons, press your thumb down on the edge of the first button, tipping the button so it stands out away from your chest.

Lay your index finger over the buttonhole for the first button. Guide the buttonhole over the up-tipped button and bring your middle finger toward the joint of your thumb, trapping the buttonhole placket between your thumb and middle finger while your thumb presses the outside edge of the button through the buttonhole and against your index finger.

Sometimes you'll see a blouse with snap fasteners. You've found a treasure!

Just as with a cuff that buttons, if you can fold the-hand-you-use small enough, by pressing your thumb against your index finger, to slide your hand through the sleeve with the cuff snap fastened that's the first option.

While the snapped cuff is less adjustable, it is more easily fastened single-handedly. You can snap the cuff for yourself by resting your forearm on a table, with the male and female sides of the snap lined up beneath your wrist. Roll your wrist so you press the snap shut between the table and your wrist.

Just as with a button-down blouse, before you start snapping up the front of the blouse, line up the shirttails in front. You don't want to snap a bunch of snaps, only to find a left over snap with nothing to snap it into on either end.

Overlay the placket of snap undersides with the placket of snap covers.

With the front and back of the first snap lined up, use your body to press the *male* end into the *female* end of each snap.

Repeat this process all the way to the bottom. Pressing the snaps together over your stomach isn't as easy as along your breastbone/sternum. It'll help to tighten your stomach muscles making a firmer background to press against.

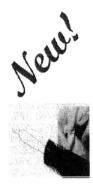

The Button Hook

When Senator Bob Dole and I spoke about the first edition of this book, his first question was *why hadn't I mentioned button hooks? Button hooks are excellent,* he insisted. I didn't discuss button hooks in the first edition of <u>One-Handed in a Two-Handed World</u> because I'd never tried one. I have now, and indeed, Senator Dole is correct. A button hook is a valuable tool.

The button hook is a stiff wire loop shaped like a pointed finger affixed to a four inch handle.

To use a Button Hook, push the wire loop of the button hook through the buttonhole you want to fasten and over the button, securing the button. Now pull the wire loop back through the buttonhole, bringing the button through too.

You may find you can help the button through the button hole by leveraging your thumb against the button. *For information on obtaining a Button Hook see* **Resources** *page 246.*

Zippered Tops, Jackets, and Coats

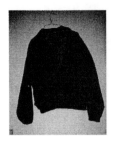

Front zippered clothing *can* be worn if you take the time to fit the *tongue* of the zipper into the zipper *slide*, trap the tongue in the slide with your middle finger and *inch-worm* zip the zipper a couple inches. Now if the zipped jacket you chose is cut loosely to allow you to pull it on and off over your head, leave it partially zipped, and wear it like a pullover.

But if it's awkward, forget it. There isn't much that looks more pathetic than someone stuck struggling with a jacket they've tried to pull on over their head.

Dresses

Back-Zip

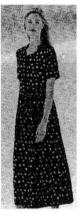

You may think you're only asking for frustration by choosing a zip up the back dress since this style isn't the easiest to operate when you have two hands.

With a little bit of planning, you can manage a back zipper as easily as a two-handed wearer. Unzip the zipper and lay the dress out on your bed back-side-up and put it on over your head just as you would a T-shirt or turtleneck (*see page* 48) With the dress on, bend over at the waist, press against a wall, trapping the dress material between your buttocks and the wall. Reach around behind and zip the zipper as high as you can, probably about mid rib somewhere. Now straighten up, so your buttocks no longer touch the wall, releasing the dress. Reach up behind your head and pull up on the neck of the dress, raising the dress until you reach the zipper handle Press your buttocks against the wall and you should be able to zip the last of the zipper up the rest of your back.

You can also choose to wear dresses that button, zip, snap, or wrap in front. If they seem a bit plain, accessorize with scarves and belts (*See **Accessories** page 63*).

Whenever possible, unbutton, unzip, or unsnap the dress, step into it, and draw your arms into the sleeves just as you would with a button down blouse (*see page 49*). Alternatively, with the top buttons, snaps, or zipper undone, put the dress on over your head, just as you would a turtle-neck or pullover top (*see page 48*). First check the tag is lined up to end up in the back, feeding the arm you don't use into it's sleeve. Follow by slipping the arm you use into it's sleeve, ducking your head into the dress, and through the neck opening.

Men

Pull-over Shirts & Sweaters

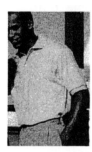

Start by laying the pull-over on the bed with the tag inside, but on top, This lines up the pull-over so you put the back over your back and the front in front.

Lift up the bottom opening and first feed the arm you don't use inside and into it's sleeve. Follow by slipping the arm you use into it's sleeve. Now, duck your head inside and with the help of your one hand, slip your head through the neck hole. Wriggle the shoulder of the hand you use to settle the pull-over shoulder onto it. Pull down on the pull-over hem all around to seat the pull-over comfortably on both shoulders and around your neck.

Taking off your pull-over single-handedly is easiest if you reach with your one hand behind your head, grab hold of your pull-over close to the neck and pull it over your head from the back. If the front neck opening gets stuck on your chin, not to worry, let go of the back and from the front ease your chin and nose through the hole, then reach back again, bringing the pull-over over your head.

Shirts

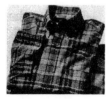

Most men's shirts fasten with buttons. There are a few things you can try to make all those buttons easier to manage. turn to page 49 for help.

Zippered Tops, Jackets, Coats

Sometimes front zipper coats and jackets *can* be done, if you take the time to fit the zipper tongue into the slide. Start the zipper a couple inches, and zip by holding the handle pinched between your index finger and thumb, and pressing your middle finger on the already zipped zipper teeth for leverage.

If the jacket is cut *roomily* enough to allow you to pull it on and off over your head, then leave the zipper zipped a couple inches and pull the jacket over your head. But it it's awkward—forget it.

Bottoms

Once you've mastered the undergarment portion of dressing your legs and lower torso (*see page 47*), handling your *public* bottom clothing isn't much different. You can benefit from a few tips on managing the extra lengths of material, and for fastening the different closures.

Women

Here, *Bottoms* refers to any clothing you wear publicly to cover your body between waist and feet. Since women have more options in this regard than do men, we'll look at mastering slacks and skirts, and kilts. (For **Dresses** *turn to page 53.*)

Slacks

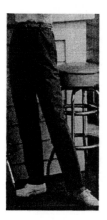

Two-handed people simply grab their slacks by the waistband one hand on either side, and hold the slacks using two hands, enabling them to step right in. Single-handedly, slacks are a bit problematic. When you hold slacks at the waistband with one hand, they don't open and it's hard to figure out where the leg openings begin, and which opening belongs to which leg.

Sit on the edge of the bed or in a chair. If the leg opposite your one hand is not affected, you'll find it's easier beginning with that leg. By stepping that *opposite* leg into the slacks, you can hold the waistband open between your one hand and that *opposite* leg. Otherwise, if the leg opposite the hand you use (*on the same side as the hand you don't use*) is affected somehow, you'll want to step into your slacks first with the leg on the same side as the hand you use. By reaching across your body with your one hand, opening the waistband, and tugging away from the one leg you've already stepped into your slacks, you can guide your opposite leg into its pant leg.

Obviously, elastic waist slacks are the easiest to manage, though slacks tend to fasten at the waist with a button.

Buttons: If the slacks you've chosen fasten with a button at the waist, you can button it single-handedly. Hook the button with your index finger and push your thumb through the buttonhole. Bring the buttonhole toward the button by pinching together your index finger and thumb.

Drag the buttonhole past the button, pulling up on the button with your index finger. Hook the buttonhole over the button by pressing with your thumb.

Snaps: To close a snap at the waist, you want to start by tightening your stomach *muscles—even if you're very thin*!

Draw the side of the waistband closure with the *male* half of the snap over your navel and hold it in place with your pinkie finger. Now, reach for the other side of the waistband closure (*the female half of the snap*) with your index finger and thumb and pinch it between those two digits, dragging the female half over the male. Now press down on the female with your index finger.

New!

Velcro: One reader of "*One-Handed in a Two-Handed World*," first edition wrote to tell me he doesn't bother with buttons, hooks or snaps at the waist of his pants. He's had all these fasteners replaced with Velcro. "*Any decent clothing store will do it for you at a nominal price*," he assured me. But you *could* do it for yourself. *For help with hand sewing, see page 161.*

Skirts

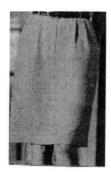

Dirndl skirts with elastic waists are no problem single-handedly. But skirts with zippers give you a more styled look. Single-handedly, you can still wear them.

Put the skirt on by stepping into it so the zipper is in front (*even if it's a back– or side–zip skirt*). Fasten the button or snap, just as described in **Slacks**, above.

To zip the zipper, face your bedroom wall, standing close enough to raise one knee and press it against the wall, trapping the skirt material just below the zipper between the wall and your knee. Trapping the skirt like this gives you leverage—like an *other* hand—allowing you to easily pull up on the zipper handle, zipping the zipper closed. Now all you need to do is pull on the waistband, dragging the zipper where it's supposed to be.

Kilts

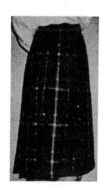

There's something so special about the way sharply pressed kilt pleats look in motion. Just because you're one-handed, doesn't mean you have to give up your kilt. Opened out, a kilt is just a long rectangular strip of material with a waistband at the top and hem at the bottom.

Put on your kilt by bending over at the waist so your back is flat. Draw the kilt across your back with the sides hanging about evenly left and right. Fasten the _inside_ waistband button or Velcro strip. Then bring the leather strap at one corner over to its buckle on the other end. Slip the tip of the strap through. You can now straighten up to fasten the buckle, or remain bent over, as you like.

Men

Trousers

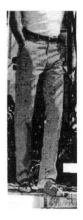

Because men's trousers pretty much always fasten at the fly, you won't need to concern yourself with more than button, snap, or slide-hook closures, and zipper. Of course, as one first edition reader suggests you can have Velcro added. (_See page 58 for details._)

"Button-flys are unnecessarily hard to manage single-handedly, so you'll want to pack up your 501s and go with zippers while you're managing single-handedly. I did years ago, with much sadness.

Two handed men grab their slacks by the waistband, one hand on either side, and hold the trousers open enabling them to step in while standing up. Single-handedly, trousers are more problematic. When you hold them by the waistband with one hand, the trousers don't open up, making it hard to figure out the leg openings—which is left and which is right.

To put on trousers single-handedly, sit on the edge of a chair. If the leg opposite your one hand is not affected, begin with that leg. After stepping that *opposite* leg into the trousers, you'll be able to hold the waistband open between your one hand and that *opposite* leg.

Otherwise, that is if the leg opposite the hand you use (*the leg on the same side as the hand you don't use*) is affected somehow, you'll want to first step into your trousers with the leg on the same side as the hand you use. Then reach across your body with your one hand to open the waistband by tugging away from the one leg already stepped into your trousers. You can now guide your *other* leg into its pant leg.

For obvious reasons, elastic waist trousers are easiest to manage single-handedly. Fear not! You can manage buttons, snaps and slide hooks one handedly.

Buttons: To fasten a button closing single-handedly, hook the button with your index finger and push your thumb through the buttonhole. Now bring the buttonhole toward the button by pinching together your index finger and thumb.

Drag the buttonhole past the button. With your index finger, lightly pull up on the button so it stands out on edge. Now hook the buttonhole over the button by pressing with your thumb.

Snaps To close a snap at the waist: Suck in your stomach, tightening the muscles. Now bring the *male* snap fitting toward the center of you, near your navel, and hold it in place with your pinkie finger. Now, with your index finger and thumb, reach for the other side of the waistband closure (*the side with the female half of the snap*) and pinch the edge of the other side of the waistband between your thumb and index finger. Draw that *other* side of the waistband closure over the first edge (*the edge trapped with your pinkie finger*). Press down with your thumb.

For **slide hook** closings, arrange the front flaps so they're close together. With your middle finger, press down on the flap with the slide. Then pinch the flap with the hook between your index finger and thumb. Still pressing down on the flap with the slide with your middle finger, lift the hook flap over the slide flap, and drag the hook over the slide. If it doesn't catch on the first pass, another try should do it.

Accessories

For both men *and* women, adding an accessory to an outfit can dress you up, or dress you down. A necktie added to a sport jacket with Dockers can get a man into a well-heeled event. Likewise, earrings, a scarf, pins, belts, etc. can transform a woman's simple outfit into elegance. Single-handedness doesn't have to reduce your fashion accessory options.

Women

Belts

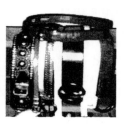

One way to dress up a simple shirt dress, a bulky sweater, or slacks and a blouse is to add a wide belt. But you already knew that... Not to worry, even single-handedly, you can still add a belt.

Bend over at the waist so your back is flat. Sling the belt over your lower back, near your waist. The buckle should hang dangling across from the belt end with the holes. Hook your thumb through the belt buckle and brace it against your stomach. Reach with your pinkie, ring, and middle fingers for the other end of the belt.

Pinch that *other end* between which ever fingers can reach it. Bring the end toward and through the buckle. Fasten the buckle and straighten up.

Scarves

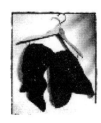

A festive scarf tied at your neck does wonders for an otherwise plain outfit. Even a gray sweatshirt has flair once you add a scarf. You may have thought unless someone else tied it for you, the bit of pizzazz from a scarf added to your outfit was lost to single-handed you. Not so! The larger square (*25" x 25"*) scarves or long rectangular strips are easiest to manage single-handedly.

Try adding loose splashes of color around your neck by: 1) folding a large square scarf in half diagonally, making a triangle. 2) pinching one of the folded corners and 3) bringing the scarf around behind you, up high enough to drop the other folded corner in front hanging over the shoulder opposite the hand you use. Now bring your hand with the other folded corner behind your head and drop that folded corner over the shoulder of the hand that you use. The folded diagonal edge of the scarf now rests along the back of your neck and the *loose* corners hang down your back between your shoulders. Bring the scarf corner you'd pinched, around under your chin, brushing past your cheek and chin. Trap that corner against your chest with your thumb

With your index and middle fingers reach for the corner you'd originally draped over the shoulder of the hand you don't use. Once you have that folded corner trapped, pinch it between your middle and ring fingers, and then, using your shoulder as leverage, between your thumb and index finger with the first corner.

Bring the pinched corners center front, under your chin. Using your lips and the hand you use, tie a loose square knot. You can choose to leave the loose corners decorating the back of your outfit, or perhaps swing them around front, or drape them over one shoulder. Play around a bit, vary the look.

* * * * *

If you need a more tailored style, instead of folding the large square scarf, just pick up the scarf by pinching one corner between your thumb and index finger. Drape it around your neck so the other end hangs over your shoulder. Draw the two ends together, one over the other, centered under your chin.

You can tie the ends using your lips and one hand, slip the ends through the ring of a scarf clip, or using a straight scarf pin, (_being careful to neither to stick your chest or to catch your blouse underneath_), to fasten the ends together. You can also fan the ends before pinning the scarf pin, or after clipping the scarf clip, or tying the ends in a simple square knot.

* * * * *

For long rectangular scarves, try tying a loose or a snug men's necktie knot. _See page 67 for tips on tying a men's necktie knot._

Alternatively, you can wrap these long scarves around your neck a couple times and then either tie a square knot with the one long end tossed casually over one shoulder, slip both ends of the scarf through a scarf clip or ring, or clip them together with a straight scarf pin.

Earrings

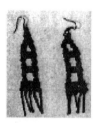

If you have pierced ears, **French Hook earrings** (*pictured left*) are the easiest to wear single-handedly. Just slide the hook through the pierced hole in your ear. Taking them out again is just as easy. Pinch the earring in front, close to your ear, and slide the hook out of the hole.

* * * * *

You *can* put on **Studs** single-handedly, but not as easily as the *French Hook* earrings. You'll want to choose stud earrings that are large and lie flat against your ear, not small ones.

To put on *studs*, you'll find it helps to tip your head to the side opposite the ear you're adorning, when you slip the post into the pierced hole. With your head tipped, gravity holds the post in place while you reach down to pick up the earring back. Now press the earring-back between your index and middle fingers closer to the pads of your fingers, with the flat side of the earring-back, the side that goes against your ear, on a plane with your index and middle finger pads—the back side of the earring back *(the clamp)* is on the same side as your fingernails. Now rest your thumb over the front of the earring that has its post already through the hole in your ear. Bring the back of the stud down onto the post sticking out behind your ear by pushing your middle and index fingers with the earring back onto the post. This takes practice.

Taking studs out of your ears involves, tipping your head back a bit, while you pinch the back between your index finger and thumb and pulling gently as you rock the earring-back, back and forth. It *will* come loose. Put down the earring back and then slip the post out of the hole by pulling forward on the earring front.

Clip-Ons are another option if *studs* prove unmanageable, and you prefer smaller close-to-your-head-style earrings than you can find with *French Hooks*.

Men

Neckties

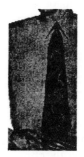

As long as men's formal business attire includes a necktie, men, with and without the use of two hands, dressing for success need to be able to manage a necktie. Not to worry, it can be done.

My grandfather Duke, (*see page 5*) easily managed his neckties after my grandmother pre-tied every new tie in a Windsor knot, leaving a loop large enough to slip the tie over his head.

All Duke's pre-knotted ties hung on the tie rack inside his closet door. Every morning, he'd select one, drop it over his head and tighten the knot by trapping the *short end* between his knee and the dresser, and sliding the knot toward his throat with his one hand. That's certainly one way to handle a necktie.

It is also possible to single-handedly tie your ties yourself. Sit down, with both feet flat on the floor. Drape the tie over your neck so the *short* end, (some 8" to 10" long) rests on your chest on the side opposite the hand you use.

Lean forward and firmly trap this *short* end between your knees. Now wrap the *long* end around the *short* end 3 times. Watch that each turn wraps smoothly (*without wrinkles or folds*). Each wrap should fall on top of the one before, and about 3" to 4" below your chin.

Now bring the *long* end of the tie up under your chin, over the front of the wraps, and under the top wrap. This forms the knot.

Pull the *long* end through until the knot is snug as well as neat and smooth.

Lastly, with the *short* end still trapped between your knees, loosely wrap your fingers around the knot and drag the knot along the *short* end up toward your chin and adjust the snugness as you like.

If neither of these ways of handling a necktie single-handedly works for you, this may be the time to explore **clip-on neckties**. They've dramatically improved in variety, and appearance. Some haberdasheries now carry clip-ons as more and more men turn to them. If yours doesn't, consider speaking with the proprietor. He may very well be able to stock clip-ons that are suitable for your wardrobe.

Tie tacks

Tie Tacks come in two pieces similar to some women's pierced earrings.

The ornamental front, has a pointed post sticking out in back and long enough to pierce through both tie tails, and the top placket of your shirt. The second piece of a Tie Tack is its back which clamps over the post point.

To put on this type of tie tack, First stand close to your dresser. Place the _Tie Tack back_ within easy reach. Pick up the front of the Tie Tack and press the post against your tie where you want to wear the tie tack.

Don't push the post through quite yet. Slide your hand to the side, resting the pad of your index finger over the front of the Tie Tack, holding it in place. But still don't push it through yet, lest the point poke through and prick your chest.

Slip your thumb underneath both ends of the tie. Between the light pressure of your index finger on the front of the Tie Tack, and your thumb, pull both ends of the tie down and away from your chest. Increase the pressure from your index finger on the front of the Tie Tack so the post pierces through both ends of the tie.

Once the post is all the way through— you can reach up with your thumb to check—the post will hold the tie tack front in the material without your holding it with your index finger. Gently let go, and pick up the *Tie Tack back* which you placed in easy reach.

Pinch the back, with the clamps on the underside, between the sides of your middle and index finger tips so the flat side of the back is parallel with the pads of those fingers. Rest your thumb on the ornamental front side of the Tie Tack. Slide the *back*, which you've clenched between your middle and index fingers, under the tie toward the point-end of the post.

By moving your thumb, angling the post, and bending your wrist, you can work the post into the hole in the T*ie Tack back.* Move your index and middle fingers, to work the clamp back over and onto the post. When you've got the two lined up, press your thumb against the ornamental front of the tie tack, pushing the post point into the Tie Tack's back clamp.

To take off your Tie Tack, reach behind your tie and squeeze the clamps in the Tie Tack back, and pull down (*toward the floor*). Then draw out the ornamental front of the Tie Tack out of your tie.

* * * * *

If this style Tie Tack doesn't work for you, look for a hinged *scissor*–style tie tack. All you do to put these on is pinch the *"scissor handles"*, and slip the *"jaws"* of the opened tie tack over and behind both ends of your tie and top placket of your shirt and release. No doubt about it, these *scissor–like* tie tacks are single-handed delights, making them *great presents for one-handed man!*

Footwear

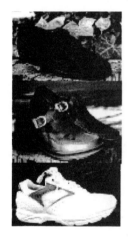

If you ever find shoes fastening with Velcro, grab them. Single-handedly speaking, NASA-developed Velcro is terrific. Regrettably, Velcro goes mainly on children's shoes, except for a few running, or leather walking shoes for adults. *For an idea of where you can locate fashionable* **Velcro Shoes**, *See* **Resources**, *Page 246.*

Not to worry! All this talk of Velcro is not to suggest that shoe laces, the old stand-by for shoes, are out of your one-handed reach. Certainly not! It's just that Velcro is infinitely easier, and shoelace tying single-handedly is different.

Women

Fashion gives women several shoe fastening options: slip-ons, buckles, gladiator straps, Velcro (*when you can find it*), and of course, laces. lip-ons, buckles and Velcro manage the same with one hand as with two.

Shoelaces

Probably the most common shoe fastener, Shoelaces require a bit of modification before they can be mastered single-handedly. Tying regular bows in your shoelaces, is a _two-handed operation._ No problem, you can still wear most your old shoes despite one-handedness.

To tie your shoes single-handedly, you first need to **re-lace your shoes**. Start re-lacing with the eyelets at the toe end of the shoe.

Thread the shoelace through the bottom-most eyelet on the side _opposite_ the hand you use, then through the other bottom-most eyelet. Don't pull the shoelace all the way through that first eyelet. Leave 6" to 8" of lace not drawn through. Thread the lace end you started with through _all_ the eyelets weaving back and forth to the top eyelet.

You should finish weaving by drawing the tip of the shoe lace through the top eyelet on the "outside" of your ankle (_your pinkie toe side_). It'll be easier to wear the off-center bow this way. (_You might want to re-lace, making sure you end up at the top eyelet in-line with your pinkie toe, though it isn't absolutely necessary._)

You need to leave about 8" of lace left over at the top. Work any excess shoelace longer than 8" back through the eyelets down to the loose end at the toe of the shoe. Knot the lace at the "_toe end_" of your shoe using a couple half hitches or the secure knot of your choice that will hold the lace firmly tied to the first eyelet at the toe of your shoe.

Cut the extra lace at the toe of your shoe. (*If it's a nylon shoelace, consider searing the cut end, to keep it from fraying.*)

Repeat this re-lacing process for your other shoe. The good news is, just like with lace-up shoes tied two-handedly, you only need to lace your shoes once—at least until you replace the laces.

To put on your shoe, first loosen the lace. After loosening the lace, you can help your shoe onto your foot by holding the shoe at the tongue to ease your toes in. Then slide your hand along the sole until you cup the heel of the shoe.

Work the shoe back and forth to seat your heel inside properly. Now tighten the shoelace so the shoe fits your foot comfortably.

You're now ready to tie this lace single-handedly. Make a 2" loop with the loose end of the shoelace (*the end extending from the top eyelet*). Slip that loop under the length of lace stretching between the top two eyelets, and then back under the piece of lace between the top eyelet and the beginning of your loop, making the knot.

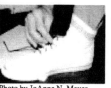
Photo by JoAnne N. Mayer

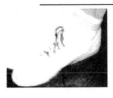

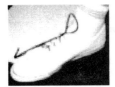

Photos by JoAnne N. Mayer

Tighten the knot by pinching the top of the loop between your index finger and thumb. Jerk the loop back and forth, first toward the same side as the arm you use and then away, two, three times.

If the knot doesn't feel tight, jerk the lace back and forth a few more times. If it *still* doesn't feel secure, you probably didn't draw the lace up through the eyelets snugly enough before starting to knot the lace. With practice, tying your shoes single-handedly will become effortless.

Promise!

To untie your shoe simply pull on the loose end of the shoe lace. Take off your shoe, by working the lace through the eyelets, loosening the lace. Cup your palm around the heel of the shoe, over the sole, and slide the shoe off your foot.

Don't worry about the *"just one loop"* in your single-handedly tied shoes. Few will notice. In more than nineteen years, the only questions have been from five or six-year-old children (*who notice everything*) and from shoe sales clerks.

Men

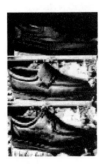

Fortunately for men, you won't be confronting as many shoe fastening options as do women. For the most part, your shoes either slip on, like loafers, or lace-up. Every once in a while you'll find a pair of casual shoes with Velcro. When you do, Buy them! Velcro's convenient.

Slipping on *loafer-like* shoes is self explanatory. Nothing to it. You just step in... If your one foot is also affected, you'll find it easier to sit down to put on your shoes and to hold the shoe by cupping the sole at the heel. Work the shoe back and forth and fit it on your foot. For help *tying lace-up shoes, see page 72.*
For ideas on finding **Velcro Shoes**, *see* **Resources**, *page 246.*

Cold-weather Clothes

There's a basic difference between the clothing you wear in cold-weather and what you wear in warm-weather—there's more of it. Cold-weather clothing also tends to fit more snugly. Clearly, you need strategies for managing all that extra snug-fitting cold-weather stuff.

Boots & Shoes

Winter snow, ice, slush, and all that stuff mean you'll need to wear boots. When you're single-handed, choosing the wrong boot reverberates all season long.

Pull-on boots tend to fit too snugly around the foot and ankle to easily slip on using one hand. Unless you find boots with some sort of expanding panel insert (*which won't be weatherproof*), pull-on boots are "*two-handed operations.*"

While you *can* re-lace boots just as you re-lace shoes, It's time-consuming to sufficiently loosen the laces allowing you to slip your foot inside, then tighten up and tie that long lacing.

Velcro would be the ultimate solution to one handable winter boots. An excellent mail-order footwear catalog with several fashionable Velcro fasten boot styles is Wissota Trader. (*See Resources page 246.*)

Zippers, another winter boot option tend to be more stylish than they are water-proof.

Coats & Jackets

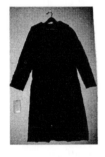

When shopping for a winter coat or parka, look for a style that doesn't zip. Sure, if the jacket is cut loosely, allowing you to leave the zipper partially zipped and be *easily* pulled over your head, you might consider it. But jackets not designed to be pulled overhead can be awkward to pull on.

There's little worse than watching a temporarily or permanently disabled someone struggle with something that doesn't work for him/her. The point of this book is helping you glide successfully single-handedly through a world designed for two-handedness.

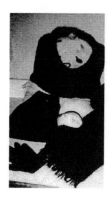

Toward that end, I strongly recommend you look for snap, Velcro, or button jacket closures all of which are conducive to graceful single-handed winters.

Shop around and you'll find styles ranging from tasteful double-breasted coats that snap or button, and perhaps with a Velcro underlay instead of a zipper. A Velcro strip used this way blocks breezes from slipping through the spaces between buttons or snaps.

Gloves & Mittens

Even in cold weather—perhaps *especially* in cold weather, your one hand must continue juggling the work of two. Because you need access to all four fingers and to your thumb in order to take advantage of the **Second Secret** (*see page11*) you need to wear a glove on the hand you use. A mitten on your one hand is far too limiting. But for your *other* hand, if you have one, for your damaged, or paralyzed fingers, or for a stump, try wearing a mitten. It's far too frustrating and time consuming to feed paralyzed, painful, or otherwise damaged fingers into a glove. A mitten for your damaged *other* hand is manageable.

If you look, you can find a mitten to almost match your one glove. You can get single gloves and mittens several ways. Buddy up with someone who uses the opposite hand and buy your gloves and mittens together. Tell your two-handed family and friends to save the one gloves and one mittens that lose their mates throughout the winter season.

Sometimes too, stores are stuck with *"orphaned"* gloves and mittens at the end of the season. Rather than paying to dispose these leftover gloves and mittens, some stores, as the weather warms, will allow you to stock up for next year at bargain prices or even *"just for the asking."*

Put the mitten on your *other hand*, first, sliding it on with the hand you use.

The first time you put the glove on your one hand, sit down. (*With practice, you'll be able to manage while standing as well.*) Lay the glove on your thigh, with the *fingers* pointing toward your knee, and the wrist opening closer to your hip.

Slide the fingers of your one hand into the opening. Brush the pads of your fingers along the bottom inside of the glove. This rubs the glove against the clothing on your *leg (slacks, skirt, overcoat, whatever...).* The friction of the glove fabric against your clothing fabric will allow you to slide your fingers into the palm area of the glove, even though the glove will slide along your thigh somewhat. Experiment.

Keep pressing down and sliding your fingers into the glove, adjusting the direction of movement so each finger lines up with the right glove finger. When your fingers are just entering the finger sections, pick up your hand and flip it over on your thigh. Now drag the back of your hand (*at this point, it should be covered by the glove cuff*) across your thigh. This will help drive your fingers deeper into the finger sections of the glove. Repeat this dragging motion of the back of your hand across your thigh a couple of times.

If your hand still isn't quite into the glove, pick up your hand and rotate it so the palm is back to resting on your thigh and rub your palm and glove across your thigh. If the hand you use still isn't yet comfortably into the glove, keep dragging your hand across your thigh, alternating between palm and the back of your hand until your glove goes on evenly, and feels right. With practice it will only take a couple passes.

Hats & Scarves

For women, the ultimate most fashionable solution to one-handed cold-weather head and neck wear is a loose-knit tube hat. It's about 22" around, and about 15" long with a thick rolled *cuff.*

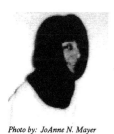

Photo by: JoAnne N. Mayer

To wear it, you pull the *not-cuffed* opening over your head until the *cuff* catches on your forehead and chin, encircling your face. The length of the tube keeps you warm by covering your head, your ears, <u>and</u> neck. It's a hat-scarf and can be a face mask all in one. If it's really cold, you can wear the *cuff* over your chin and covering your face.

More convenient yet, once you get to your destination, you can simply slip the cuff down behind your head to the nape of your neck so the tube rings your neck like a cowlneck—Black compliments most any cold weather outfit—long after you've arrived, even if you stay indoors.

By wearing your tube hat, even while inside, you aren't confronted with the awkwardness of peeling off a hat, scarf, and coat, a glove, and mitten, and perhaps even boots, in the front hall—all single-handedly while trying to keep everything together—then trying to find it all again, to reassemble yourself when it's time to leave. With a tube hat, you never have to take off and risk losing, your hat *and* scarf. You wear it out, and don't take it off 'til you're back home.

* * * * *

You can also wear off-the-shelf knitted wool caps. Loosely woven styles are easiest to manage single-handedly.

Fold the hem, making a cuff, and then pick up the hat by the back. Spread the sides of the hat open by stretching the whole length of your hand—thumb to wrist—along the inside of the cuff. Roll the rest of your fingers over the material, pressing them into your thumb.

Tip your head forward and pass the loose cuff of the hat against your forehead, until the cuff front catches on your forehead. Draw the back cuff down over the *point* of your head, sliding the back of the hat over the back of your head.

Let go of the back cuff of the hat. Now stretch your thumb and middle finger apart in a wide "V," and press them against the hat so they straddle your forehead. Draw the hat down on your forehead and in back, by dragging your thumb and middle finger "V" in the front, and in the back with the palm of your hand.

* * * * *

You can also wear off-the-shelf wool scarves single-handedly. There's really no need to knot a scarf to reap the warmth of a scarf around your neck. A scarf smoothly wrapped around is just as warm, and far more flattering.

Try it this way: Start one end of the scarf so it lies across your chest. Now draw the other end around your neck and drop that end across your chest, making an "X" with the first end.

Smooth any wrinkles in the scarf against your neck. With the two ends lying flat on your chest, You have layers of scarf at your throat and on your chest. You also have a layer of scarf around your neck and under your coat collar.

With a long wide scarf, try it *Babushka* style so your head too, instead of just the back of your neck is covered as are your throat and your chest, by that same strip of wool. Do just as described above, but instead of drawing the scarf around your neck, drape it over your head, the ends dropping down at your ears, wrap the ends, one at a time, under your chin, leave whatever is left of each end draped across your chest.

Warm-weather Clothes

Warm-weather clothes are easier to manage single-handedly than those worn in cold-weather. Not only because there are fewer of them, but because there's less to them, they're lightweight, and loose-fitting styles more comfortable in warm weather, are more easily managed.

You've already seen that an ample sleeve width, for that *"other" arm and shoulder* is an important consideration when selecting tops (*see page 49*). It's probably already obvious to you how looser styles, in lighter-weight fabrics make single-handed comfortable and attractive dressing easier yet.

Bathing caps

Most swimming pools require bathing caps on every head: male, female and child. It no longer matters how short you wear your hair. So you'll need a strategy to single-handedly master bathing caps. *Swim team caps* are the easiest for one-handers. You put a bathing cap on much the same as you put on your knit cap all winter (*see page 79*). Spread the sides of the bathing cap open by putting the whole length of your thumb, to your wrist inside the *"hem"* band along the back of the cap.

Roll the rest of your fingers into the cap by pressing your knuckles against the palm of your hand, so you're holding the hem of the bathing cap between your palm and the pads of your fingers. Tip your head forward and drag the front *hem* of the cap over the point of your head until it catches on your forehead. Now draw the back of the cap down onto the back of your head. Position the cap comfortably on your head by stroking it with your thumb and middle finger, spread in a wide "V," in the front and using the flat of your hand in the back.

Bathing suits

Women

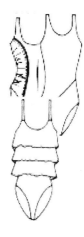

Women have a number of considerations when choosing swimwear. Not only do we need to like the color, but there's the pattern, whether it fits well— flattering our figures. And now that you're one-handed, whether you can get into it...

No wonder it's hard to find a satisfactory bathing suit! One-handers want to avoid any suit with straps tying behind the neck. You'd have to find someone else to take care of the tying unless the suit you've chosen that ties behind your neck, allows you to step in and out when left tied.

One-piece competition-style swim suits (*like what Olympic women swimmers wear*), now available in fabulous colors, patterns, and designs, fill the bill for easy single-handed access, style, originality, and figure flattery. Watch out for complicated strap arrangements though. Straps interwoven across your back—although they do look sharp—are difficult to figure out single-handedly, when it comes to getting into the suit.

Men

For guys, other than color, fabric, and patterns, your swimwear choices range from racing briefs to trunks. Once you've mastered your boxer shorts or jockey briefs, (*see page 47*) you shouldn't have a problem.

Footwear

When warm weather finally arrives, it's tempting to kick-off your sensible, sturdy shoes, and head for the sandals or even to bare down to flip-flops. If you're newly, or temporarily one handed, do think twice about that urge.

Arms and hands are closely integrated with maintaining balance while you're upright. It may take some months to get used to the changes one-handedness makes to your equilibrium. If you're still getting used to the changes in your equilibrium, now is not the time to complicate matters with non-supportive flimsy shoes.

While you're in the early stages of one-handedness, you want to choose your summer shoes carefully. Look for arch support in the sole, sufficient straps to secure the shoe onto your foot, and buckle or Velcro closures. You'll need to invest extra time this year looking for your warm weather footwear. But if you don't make that investment you may wish you had, especially if you fall and re-injure your _other_ hand or arm, or worse yet, the one hand you _can_ use.

What to avoid

Women, as it gets warmer, you may consider trading-in your heavier _"Sheer-Energy"_ panty hose (_See page 45_) for those so-called _summer sheers_. **_Don't do it._** You'll only rarely succeed in pulling on sheer hose single-handedly. Inevitable you'll poke one or all your four fingers right through ruining a new pair of pantyhose when you don't have time.

It's not worth the frustration. Besides sheers aren't much cooler anyway. Nylon on your legs is nylon on your legs. You'll probably be going from air conditioning to air conditioning anyway.

Be sure to avoid: tops that button *up the back,* and front-zippered tops that aren't roomy enough to easily slip over your head with the zipper partially closed.

Look for Snaps, Buttons or Velcro.

You'll also want to watch out for ***drawstrings***, a popular styling accent for warm-weather fashions. Drawstrings are difficult to single-handedly tie securely or attractively enough.

EATING

At first, facing three or more utensils, all needing to be somehow manipulated single-handedly presents an almost over-whelming challenge. This challenge may be even further complicated depending upon how it was you became one-handed.

If you experienced a head injury or perhaps a stroke, you may also be dealing with *secondary* deficits like **hemianopsia** (*peripheral vision blindness*), **spatial disorientation** *(where you are in relation to other things)*, or perhaps poor **propioception** *(awareness of where affected limbs are (often a problem following traumatic brain injury or stroke*).

Each *secondary* deficit adds new complications to single-handed eating. The first step to successful coping is knowing about secondary effects from the injury causing your one-handedness. Discuss this with your OT (*Occupational Therapist.*)

Not to worry though, even single-handedly, you can learn to eat as gracefully as the most refined two-handed diner, so elegantly and efficiently that even the venerable Madam's Post and Manners would and would approve.

As if just mastering all those utensils weren't enough, there are also unique and sometimes unexpected challenges to resolve when eating away from home.

For example, in restaurants you'll be confronted with individual serving-size plastic butter, jelly and coffee creamer tubs, with footed dessert bowls designed to be held with one hand while one digs into the densely packed food such as ice cream or sherbet, and with buffet tables laden with dozens of dishes from which one is to serve him/herself.

There *are* ways to manage each of these situations single-handedly. *See pages 112—butter tubs, 96—ice cream in a cup and 113—buffet tables, to skip ahead for details.*

Beverages

Soda

At first glance, it may have seemed that opening a can of soda one handedly would be no problem. After all, all you have to do is _flip_ the top...

Bu-ut, then when you rashly reached for the can, to flip that top—if you were unfortunate—too late you realized that two-handed people have an _other_ hand to hold the can steady while flipping the top with the index finger on the one hand. When you first try single-handedly, your partially open can most likely tipped over, spilling soda all over.

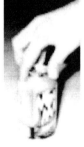

To successfully open a flip-top soda can single-handedly, set the soda can on a table (_with practice, even when there's no table available, you'll learn to rest the soda can on your thigh_). Leverage the can by pressing your index and ring fingers and thumb against the rim, across from each other (_pictured, left_). Now, with the can leveraged, try flipping the top open prying the ring with your middle finger.

Photo by JoAnne N. Mayer

Tea

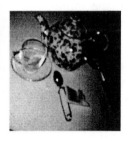

Obviously, tea bags are wonderfully one-handable. Still and all, loose tea steeped free of the paper bag truly _does_ taste better. Tea balls are <u>not</u> one-handable.

To make tea from loose tea leaves, single-handedly, add a **Tea Infuser** to your kitchen gadgetry. Tea Infusers operate like tongs with a basket at the end to hold the loose tea. Scissor open the "_baskets_" and plunge them into the loose tea canister.

Don't over pack tea leaves into the basket. Boiling water needs to caress the leaves to steep properly.

Alternatively, you can choose to drop a *pinch* of loose tea directly into your tea-pot, and, with a sieve over each teacup as you pour steeped tea out of the pot, strain the tea from the loose tea leaves.

Wine

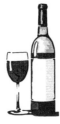

Even single-handedly, it's nice, to be able to open the wine *for* your guests—*for* yourself. You *can*! Just remember that some cork screws manage more easily than others.

You don't want to struggle with a bare bones, basic cork screw, the kind that simply screws into the cork using pure brute strength to twist in, and with even more brute force, is hauled out corkscrew and cork together.

Single-handedly, you'll manage more gracefully if you use a **winged corkscrew** (*pictured left*).

To open your bottle of wine, first cut away the foil-plastic seal covering the cork by scraping a knife across the top of the cork and against the bottle rim.

Place the bottle between your thighs, cork facing out and angled about 75° toward the ceiling, holding it with your adductor muscles.

Press the tip of the cork screw against the center of the cork, and begin twisting it into the cork.

As the corkscrew digs into the cork with your twisting, the *cuff*, in accordance with its design, fits over the wine bottle rim, settling onto the rim, and pulling against the cork with every twist on the cork screw, thus beginning to draw the cork out of the bottle.

The *winged* lever arms on your cork screw rise, spreading out as you twist the cork screw deeper into the cork. Keep twisting until the lever arms (wings) are about a 45° angle to the bottle.

Now, with your thumb and pinkie finger (*or ring finger if your hand spread is large enough*) pull the lever arms (the *wings*) down, parallel with the corkscrew, drawing the cork part-way out of the bottle with minimal effort. When the *wings* are parallel with the cork screw, the cork will either be all the way out, or close enough that a light tug on the corkscrew will pull out the cork.

* * * * *

Pump corkscrews also work well single-handedly. You simply plunge the hollow syringe-like prong, into the wine cork. As you pump the handle, you force air into the wine bottle. This air pushes the cork out. The pump corkscrew has at least two advantages: 1) You'll rarely lose cork debris into the wine, and 2) your guests will be impressed by this gadget.

Breads

It's all the rage: breads served European-style—unsliced loaves in wicker baskets and kept warm under a freshly ironed linen cloth. Each diner is expected to take the bread in *both hands* and tear away a serving.

Sometimes you'll find one of your dining companions has torn off twice as much as s/he meant to. Usually, that over-sized serving gets torn in half, and the extra returned to the basket. Whenever this happens, your problem of managing unsliced bread single-handedly has been resolved for you. You only need take the broken away bread left behind by this dining companion.

When you must break away your own serving single-handedly, try not to be the first to break into the loaf. Let a two-handed someone else tear into the loaf first since that first piece is the hardest to break off with one hand, especially with a thick crust bread.

When it's your turn to tear away a serving, bring the bread close to you, and keep the *Second Secret* in mind (*see page* 12). If your main course hasn't arrived, place the basket in front of you. Reach into the basket, and take hold of the loaf straddling your thumb and middle finger around it. Stretch your index finger out to where you want to tear off the bread and press your index finger down into the loaf.

With your thumb and middle finger pinching the bread you want, pull up and away-from your index finger. The bread will begin to tear, but you won't probably be able to break off your piece yet.

That's okay. Stop pulling when the tearing stops and flip the loaf over. Grab hold of the up-side-down loaf just as you held it before, between your thumb and middle finger.

Don't forget to stretch out your index finger again, pressing down it into the loaf. With your thumb and middle finger, pull up and away from your index finger. When the bread stops tearing, pull away your serving.

Buttering Bread

In the hospital, the staff will use your knife to butter toast for you. After leaving the hospital, your well-meaning friends will still do the same, but not forever—and they're not always available.

It's one thing to butter toast for everyone at the table, and quite something else, for someone to lean over and take toast off an adult's plate and butter it. The first is polite while the second feels patronizing.

Just because you're one-handed doesn't mean you can't butter your own bread, or spread your own jelly, jam, cream cheese, peanut butter, etc. This method following works with bread, toast, bagels, hard breads, and even rice cakes.

It works on just about anything you'd want to spread butter/margarine/ cream cheese/peanut butter/jelly on. Maybe even for spreading glue or putty! Bottom line rule, as always. Your imagination's the key to managing single-handedly. If an idea looks like it might work, it probably will, with adaptation(s).

Slicing butter/margarine away from the stick in a butter dish, or taking enough cream cheese from the aluminum foil wrapped package isn't a problem.

You'll want use a butter dish—*No more saucers. (The stick invariably fits edge-to-edge in a saucer and saucers are convex. As you cut down on the stick of butter, the pressure on your butter knife rocks the saucer. Single-handedly, you have no other hand to hold things steady. So, save yourself the aggravation, and use a butter dish.)*

To *spread* the butter/margarine/ jelly/cream cheese or whatever, hold your knife by wrapping your fingers around the handle with the blade at a 45° angle to the toast and rest the knife blade against the pile of butter.

Trap the toast with your thumb. Now pull the knife toward you, by closing your fingers into a fist. This way you drag whatever you want to spread across your toast—spreading it.

To spread the butter more evenly, simply turn the toast. Maybe once, maybe two, three times. With practice, this method looks efficient, even easy; and far better than the scrape-scrape process two-handed people use.

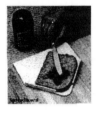

If you can't get this method using *"body positioning"* to work for you, ask your OT (*Occupational Therapist*) about a **Spreading Board** [*pictured left*]. It's designed to hold your slice of bread steady while you spread the whatever. *For information on obtaining a **Spreading Board** See* **Resources** *page 246.*

Dessert

Once you've figured out how to manage main courses single-handedly, it's a relief to find Desserts: cakes, cookies, most candies, pies, cakes, etc. are infinitely *single-handable* if you keep in mind the helpful hints provided below *"Soft Food on a Flat Plate"* (*See page 104*). By creatively manipulating your fork, you'll effortlessly finesse the delightful, sweeter courses.

Ice cream

Cones

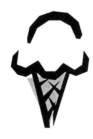

While you lick your one-handable ice cream cone, your one hand is unavailable for anything else—including wiping a napkin across your lips. All the same, ice cream cones are most manageable single-handedly. *Remember to pay for your cone before the clerk hands it to you. Count out the cost while it's being scooped, and set the money on the counter. Otherwise you'll have the awkward experience of handing the cone back to the startled clerk—usually a high school student—while the folks in line behind you shuffle around irritably as you fumble for money.*

Dishes

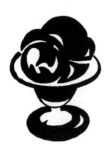

Adapt the method for managing slices of melon (*see page 99*) as described below, to successfully handle a dish or take-out cup of ice cream. You do *not* always have to order ice cream in a cone!

Pick up the spoon, holding it with your fingers wrapped around the handle halfway down the shaft. The *"shovel-end"* (*or bowl of the spoon*) will be at a 90º angle to the ice cream.

Rest the bowl of the spoon on edge of the on the ice cream. Align your thumb against the side of the cup. The purpose of your thumb here, is to hold the cup steady as you dig into the ice cream for a bite-sized serving. Dig the spoon into the ice cream by pulling your knuckles toward your palm, tightening your fist, and scooping into the ice cream.

Ta-da.

You now have a bite-sized scoop of ice cream in the bowl of your spoon! To get that scoop gracefully into your mouth; Keeping the spoon level, loosen your fingers, allowing the spoon handle to slide down your fingers until it rests on your index finger pad. Now rest your thumb on the handle and pinch the handle between your index finger and thumb. Bring the butt end of the spoon through the opening between your middle finger and thumb, with your index finger's help. Now look. You're holding your spoon just the way Emily Post said you should!

Savor, and then, go ahead, do it again.

Fruits & Vegetables

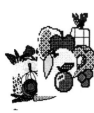

Eaten raw, most fruits and vegetables are infinitely *one-handable*. Choices known as *"finger food"* are intended to be picked up with the fingers of one hand— but you already figured that out, right?

Bananas

They're known as "the *perfect food.* But not so perfect, you might say, as you contemplate a banana single-hand-edly. Use your cutting board (*see page 120*) to score the stem end of the skin. Then, leaving your banana lying on the cutting board or resting on a plate, peel away the skin section-by-section. You may find it more comfortable to eat your banana using a plate and fork after you've peeled the skin from your banana, and tossed the skin in the garbage.

Grapefruit

Prepare grapefruit for breakfast with the help of your *cutting board* (*see page120*). Impale the grapefruit on the cutting board nails so your sharp serrated knife slices between the nails when you cut the grapefruit in half, and cuts across the grapefruit sections. Pick each grapefruit half off your cutting board. Select one, and impale it on your cutting board, skin side down, fruit side up. Now, with a steak knife or, if you have one, a true grapefruit knife, slice the sections, cutting between the section membrane and the pulp meat of the fruit. Then, with an up and down sawing motion, cut around the inside of the outside skin, separating it from the fruit.

Try serving grapefruit to yourself in a cereal bowl (*The sides make scooping the fruit easier*). You may find *Dycem* (*see page 129*) or a plastic place mat under your bowl helps add traction.

Melon

As a kid, it fascinated me when my grandmother served melon. She festively refilled our wedges with -sized balls of melon—what a marvelously playful way for us kids to eat melon. We simply pricked the balls with forks.

It wasn't until I was older that my mother explained; melon balls were a device Gram used enabling my grandfather, Duke, (*see page 5)* to easily enjoy melon after he lost his hand.

But you don't have to resort to a melon baller   to enjoy melon single-handedly. The first post-hemorrhage melon I faced, frustrated me so much I wasn't sure whether I wanted to cry or throw it at someone. I was sure everyone saw me struggling with the damn thing, and was laughing, or worse yet, feeling sorry for me. That melon was served on a flat dessert plate and tastefully decorated with a sliver of orange, a sprig of parsley and three grapes. The melon balanced evenly on its rind, right in front of me, like a pastel orange grin.

It looked so good. I could almost taste its scent. I'd picked up my spoon, (*Dad always told me melon was properly eaten with a spoon.*) and had proceeded to dig into the tip closest to the hand I use. Melons tend to be juicy, and naturally, this one was no exception. As I poked at it with my spoon, the melon rocked sliding around my plate, away from my spoon.

Since I couldn't grab the thing with my one hand and cut into it with the spoon at the same time, or trap it with a fork, like some of my dining companions were, I was out of luck. Even tipping the wedge over on it's side didn't work. It still skidded around the plate every time I tried to spoon-cut a piece.

It was a rather formal affair, and neither the time nor the place to experiment with single-handling solutions, so I just pushed the plate away, and waited for the next, *hopefully more manageable,* course.

While living with my folks, post-hemorrhage, Mom used to prepare melon for me by separating the melon fruit from its skin with a knife and slicing the fruit into bite-sized chunks.

You *can* eat melon without waiting for someone to prepare it. Using your cutting board (*see page 120*) fix a melon for yourself, for breakfast maybe.

Impale the melon on the nails. Slice the whole melon in half. Now cut each half in half by turning the *cut*-side (*flat-edge*) of each down on the cutting board, so the melon's skin-side up (*this stabilizes the melon so you won't need to impale it on the nails again—a bit of a time-saver*), now slice.

If you want, you can cut the quarter slices in half again. Just impale each quarter slice on the cutting board nails and slice. Once you have the serving sizes of your choice (*quarter, eighth slices*) one at a time impale each, with the nails protruding near the center (*measuring tip to tip*) of the slice and, starting from one tip, slide the knife between the skin and the melon fruit. Repeat this cut from the other tip. Once the fruit is separated from the skin, cut the fruit into bite-sized chunks.

Oranges

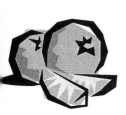

You may have thought you could no longer enjoy an orange unless it came in a can or it was peeled for you. Not so! With your cutting board's help (*see page 120*) you can fix oranges for your self!

Impale the orange on your cutting board so the nails straddle the navel. Using a serrated knife cut the orange in half. Pull the halves off the nails. Laying the halves on the cutting board, cut side down, slice each in half.

You may be tempted—after all this time without tasting an orange you prepared for yourself—to bite into the whole orange quarters just the way they are, while standing over the kitchen sink, the juice dribbling down your chin and into the sink. Oranges taste great that way!

But if you're serving company, or you feel like sitting down and more decorously enjoying your orange, cut each quarter cross-wise, in thirds, making orange chunks with a bit of rind on each chunk. The rind is perfect for holding onto when you bite into the orange fruit.

Tossed Salad

Once you learn this trick for managing wooden salad utensils single-handedly, you'll find you also easily manage chopsticks at Chinese restaurants—even rice! So use the chopsticks even at a table also set with Western flatware.

Pick up both serving utensils together, half way down the handles, just as you'd hold a pen, and so that the fork tines and the spoon bowl press together. Slip your middle finger between the handles so the top handle, either spoon or fork, is pinched between your index and ring fingers, and resting on your thumb. The bottom utensil is pinched between your pinkie and ring fingers and pressed into the webspace between your thumb and index finger by the length of your thumb. Operate the top utensil by pressing and relaxing your index finger.

* * * * *

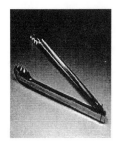

A quick and easy solution for serving tossed salad to yourself while at the table is to use your stainless steel kitchen tongs—the same ones you use to pick hot corn on the cob, asparagus, or lobster out of the pot.

If you look, you can find decorative tongs more suitable for the dining room table than the utilitarian-style kitchen tongs pictured to the side, but in a pinch, these will do the trick.

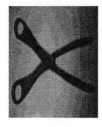

* * * * *

Another option is a ***wooden scissor-tong***. This is infinitely single-handed and far more tasteful for the dining table than are your kitchen tongs. It's so easy to use, and good-looking you might even start a trend among your friends.

Main Courses

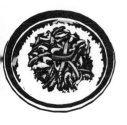

By remembering to keep ease of consumption in mind when you choose your main course, you'll save yourself from ordering sirloin steak on the one night you've forgotten to bring your Rocker knife (*see page 109*) to the restaurant with you.

Manageable Foods

When planning your meals, plan foods that easy to eat, but don't forget to factor in a well-rounded healthy diet. In the sections that follow you'll find suggestions to help you with foods that at first might not seem to fall into the *"easy-to-eat"* category, but with modification to your approach become infinitely doable.

Easy to eat main courses include most vegetarian entrees, fish, fowl (*chicken, duck, goose, and turkey, for example*). For your red meat, consider meatloaves, beef stew, corned beef, or tender pot roast, hearty soups, stews, and goulashes, etc.

Truly though, as long as you have the accessories and gadgets you need, you can pretty much eat what you like. Some foods are just easier.

Soft Foods on a Plate

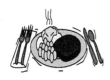 Two-handed people simply push food onto their fork by trapping it between the fork and a knife held in their *other* hand. Since there isn't an *other* hand for you, you'll have to improvise.

Try using other food on your plate as walls to push against. Foods like baked potatoes, broccoli, asparagus, and meat patties make good barriers. Try spearing with your fork, anything *spearable*. peas, lima beans, broccoli and cauliflower florets, chunks of meat, and chunks of fruit. This tactic makes a number of different foods single-handedly manageable.

Inevitably though, you'll sit down to a meal with an abundance of soft foods, like mashed potatoes, hash, peas, gelatin, rice. don't worry, you can handle these meals.

Hold your fork with your fingers wrapped around the handle, far down the stem—your index finger as close to the prongs as possible and your thumb resting against the prong closest to you. When holding your fork this way, as you open up your fist, the fork will be at a right angle to your plate. As you tighten your fist, the fork flattens, parallel to your plate. Practice, and you'll see.

Loosen your fist, the fork is at a 90° angle, and position the prongs behind the food you wish to eat. Rest the side prong against your plate. Stretch out your thumb at a right angle to your palm, resting it on your plate, in front of the bite-sized amount of food you want to scoop onto your fork.

This way, your thumb is the "*wall*" you needed to push against. With the fork at a right angle behind the food and your thumb in front, tighten your fingers into a loose fist, drawing the fork under that bite of food and toward your thumb, flattening the fork so that it slides under the food.

Now, loosen your hold on the fork and rest the prong end on your plate. The handle should be cradled on your middle finger. Slide that middle finger along the handle, stopping about an inch and a half before the end.

Press the fork handle between your index finger and your thumb. Your thumb and index fingers form an opening over the fork butt end. Bring the butt end of the fork through that opening by lowering your palm toward the table and simultaneously pushing the butt end through the opening with your middle finger.

The butt end of the fork now rests against your index finger between the first and second knuckles and you're holding your fork just the way Miss Manners instructs, and that bite of food is still on the tines of your fork, ready for you to lift toward your mouth normally!

At first, this procedure may seem cumbersome, but with practice, it becomes quick and smooth, even graceful.

For added stability on the plate end of this process, lay some Dycem (*see page 129*) on the table beneath your dinner plate, or use a plastic-coated place mat.

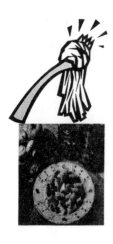

Pasta

Long thin spaghetti pasta is the most difficult to manage single-handedly, without a spoon held in an *other* hand to against which to twirl your selected forkful . Just "*twirling*" against your plate doesn't segregate a mouthful of spaghetti. You'll always end up with long dangling ends slapping red sauce on your chin and neck.

If you must eat spaghetti single-handedly, you can try cutting the spaghetti into more manageable lengths and use the procedure described for eating soft foods on a dinner plate (*see page 104*). Or you can try segregating a *manageable* amount on your plate (*5 or 6 strands*) and twirl it around the prongs of your fork. You'll inevitably need to contend with the ends that won't stay twirled.

The most effective pasta solution is to stay away from spaghetti when you're one-handed, and to order "*spearable*" pasta like **Ziti** (*with or without lines*), **Rotini** (*spirals*), **Shells**, or **Farfalloni** (*bow ties*), for example. These pasta shapes allow you to competently arrange appropriately-sized mouthfuls of food on your fork.

Staying neat

One of the keys to eating independently, is looking as though you're managing everything just fine. One way to look as though you're managing everything just fine, is to stay neat—or at least to organize things so your clothing isn't soiled by the food you're eating.

Napkins

When you first start eating single-handedly, and for a while after that, you'll find eating can be a messy business. All your upper body movement tends to be with the one side you use, and inevitably the napkin you so carefully spread across your lap will have fluttered to the floor unnoticed by you, so when one of those slips *"twixt the cup and the lip"* happens, it falls smack dab in the middle of your unknowingly unprotected lap.

If you take special care to anchor a corner or two of your napkin under you, your apkin'll stay put better.

Alternatively, children don't have to be the only ones with napkins tucked into their shirt collars. You'll only look ridiculous when you don't and you're spending the rest of the evening with food stains all over the front of your clothing.

Bibs

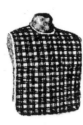

Where I come from (*My hometown is North of Boston, MA.*) lobster, served in its shell piping hot and bright red, is a favorite, but messy with a capital "M" entree. Whenever one prepares to eat lobster with anyone else at the table, s/he first dons a *"lobster bib."* Many of the first-class restaurants specially design souvenir lobster bibs available for purchase at the register as diners leave still savoring their meal. Long bibs with *Velcro* closings also covering the lap, are the only attire appropriate for eating a lobster dinner.

Just as cooks wear aprons when cooking, you can choose to wear a bib whenever dining with company. *Catchy "designer"-styled bibs make terrific Christmas gifts*—even better than the ties and mugs people usually give, because they've truly been selected with *you* in mind.

Utensils

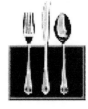

With some minor alterations in the way you hold each utensil (*see pages 96, 93, 104, for example*) and some practice, you can learn to use regular flatware; forks, spoons, and knives. It's a fact however, that cutting "tough foods like red meat, single-handedly won't happen if you just try using a steak knife.

If meat is a staple of your diet, or even if you enjoy eating it once-in-a-while, you'll need an adapted cutting knife. You'll want to bring this adaptive knife (*See suggestions below.*) with you when you dine out so you won't need to prevail on someone else to cut the meat *for* you. There are variations on knife adaptations which accommodate both your one wrist's strength and your use preferences.

Rocker knife

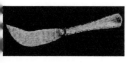

Designed with a sharp curved blade, and in a variety of handle styles, the Rocker Knife allows you to cut your foods by rocking the blade front to back, rather than by sawing. The *rocking* motion means you don't need an *other* hand to anchor what you're cutting.

"Cut-Up Knife"

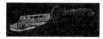

The **Cut-Up knife** is a *higher-tech* version of the Rocker Knife. The serrated blade in a jointed base combines pressure with the rocking allowing you to cut your food with less pressure from your wrist.

DINING OUT

Whenever you go out to eat, you'll want to bring with you your rocker knife (*see page 109*), your stylish bibs (*see page108*), and any other helpers you use when eating at home. This way, you can be an equal member at the table and your dining companions won't feel the need to help you with your dinner.

Alternatively, you can try advising your waiter that your main course—if it requires cutting—needs to be cut in the kitchen for you. Some waiters are amenable to such special requests. Others belabor the point, turning a simple request into an embarrassment. Embarrassing to you, and to your dining companions. So, remembering to bring the gadgets with which you've become accustomed, when eating away from home can help ensure dining out is the pleasant experience it's supposed to be.

Individual butter tubs

Let's start **Dining Out** by looking at those *"cute"* single serving tubs, the ones with foil covers used by restaurants, and with take-out food. The packaging for butter, margarine, jellies, and cream. When you first try managing these things single-handedly, they're daunting. Especially, if you go at them directly and try scooping at the *whatever* with your knife. There is an easier way.

Peel the aluminum cover back by holding the tab between your thumb and index finger and resting your middle finger on the tub edge. Your middle finger holds the tub steady while you pull the aluminum foil lid. Then, turn the tub up-side-down over the toast, holding it on the long sides between your thumb and middle finger, pinch the tub at the edges. Rest your index finger along the bottom of the tub. Pull up on the sides with your thumb and middle finger, pressing down with your index finger. This way you'll turn the tub inside out, forcing its contents onto your toast with your index finger pressed against the tub bottom.

For help with spreading what you've gotten out of the tub, s*ee page 93.*

Buffets, & Salad Bars

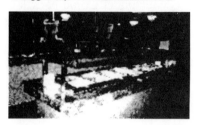

To easily accommodate single-handed patrons, buffets, salad bars, and cafeterias need to be designed more effectively. Two-handed patrons would be better served too. My wish list includes things like a *"raceway tray shelf"* all around the perimeter of the buffet table for sliding your tray along, *enough space* between the selections to rest your dish while serving yourself, *lighter plates*, lighter and sturdier trays, and *space under the coffee spigot that's deep enough to set down your cup* while you fill it and that has some sort of drainage so the bottom of your coffee cup stays dry and clean.

Although restaurants and restaurant supply houses haven't yet heard my wish list, you need not forgo the buffet/salad bar/cafeteria *all-you-can-eat* extravaganzas while you're one handed. Try these ideas.

If there isn't a *tray shelf* around the perimeter, roll your flatware into a napkin and stuff the package into your pocket.

Leave enough of it showing so it's obvious you're not trying to sneak out of the place with restaurant property. Don't use a tray at all. Just go through the buffet holding your plate. Come back later for your beverage, and dessert if you're so inclined.

If everything's tightly crammed onto the buffet table, the good news is it's probably jam-packed with delicacies. The bad news is it'll be a little more difficult to serve yourself single-handedly.

More difficult yes, but by no means impossible. Most of the selections will be in bowls of smaller diameter than your plate. All you need to do is set your plate on top of one bowl while you serve yourself from others. Salad dressing bowls tend to be particularly good for this purpose. Alternatively, if the serving bowls are set closely together, you can often set down your plate by resting it over the sides of three adjacent bowls.

Heavy ceramic plates are only really problematic if you choose to use a tray. Otherwise, with flatware in your pocket, you need only carry the plate, so it shouldn't be too heavy alone.

Sometimes there's a spill-tray grate directly below the coffee urn spigot. Inevitably, though, the clearance between that grate and the spigot is half an inch too low to slide your cup in straight on. That means you can't set down your cup on the grate and fill it full because you'll have to tip the cup to the side to work it out from beneath the spigot. That's okay for those who add cream or milk afterwards, but for those of us who like a full cup of black Java, it's darn annoying.

If there's nothing but open air, and a wastebasket to catch the dribbles, below the coffee urn spigot, usually the case at community events where they give you a small Styrofoam cup. You can still manage. Pinch the cup between your index and middle fingers with your index finger inside the cup, but only as deep as the end of your cuticle or beginning of the first knuckle. Twist your hand around so the cup is under the spigot, and reach up to pull down on the spigot handle with your thumb. It's a bit of a stretch, but *can* be done. *Careful you don't fill the cup too full. You don't want to burn your one index finger.* Once again, you won't get a full cup, but mostly full sure beats none.

Fun Food & Snacks

Yes, of course you can enjoy snack foods single-handedly. Even the kind of snacks you're supposed to reach in for a handful, munch until that handful is consumed, and then reach in for some more—for instance, popcorn:

Popcorn

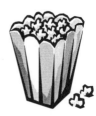

You might not think of popcorn as a *two-handed* snack, especially when you're eating out of your own bowl on a table next to you. But if you're sharing a bowl that's circulating—and it's a while between rotations, you'll want to take more than a couple kernels; when you're at someone's house, or in a movie theater, there won't be any place to lay down a handful so you can pick one popped kernel at a time and eat it.

Not to worry, you can still get your share. When the bowl comes around, pass it to the next person and while they hold it, dig in taking a handful. To eat the popcorn, bring the handful to your face. Delicately touch the tip of your tongue against a kernel of popcorn. It'll stick to the moisture on your tongue, allowing you to draw the kernel into your mouth. Chew, and swallow. Don't worry, no one will notice how you're doing this, because your hand, and the popcorn in it hide your tongue darting out to catch popcorn pieces.

Unshelled Peanuts

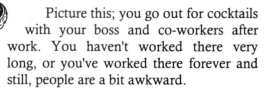

Picture this; you go out for cocktails with your boss and co-workers after work. You haven't worked there very long, or you've worked there forever and still, people are a bit awkward.

They pick the bar. Maybe it's kind of a folksy, comfortable place, macramé curtains in the windows, raw beams overhead, hardwood floors, and wooden ladder-back chairs with caned seats around heavy, round, maple tables. The ceiling fans spin lazily overhead swirling cigarette smoke. Easy listening love songs play on the jukebox, a little too loudly. Your group picks a table, sits down, and orders drinks. The table is set with a single red carnation in a clear cut glass vase, a heavy amber glass ashtray, and a wicker basket full of unshelled peanuts. Aha!

Or perhaps it's a rowdy after work pub, rock-and-roll—Beatles blare from a jukebox. Navy blue, gray, and brown pinstripe suits line the bar.

Everyone carries a bright frozen drink, the margaritas distinguished only by salt on the glass and lack of umbrella. They're all bellied up to the bar, talking shop. You sit down, in front of the glass bowl of unshelled peanuts.

* * * * *

Pick out an unshelled peanut and proceed to _unshell_ it, but not the usual way. You'll not shatter the shell in fragments.

Hold the peanut at the seams, between your thumb, index, and middle fingers. Squeeze firmly, but not so hard the shell shatters, just firmly enough to split the seam at the _not-stem end_. As soon as the seam separates, slide the tip of your index finger nail and finger into the split gently splitting the peanut shell in half along the seams.

At this point, you may find it helpful to rest the *stem end* (*the not-split end*) on the table or bar for added leverage. Pull the shell apart between your index finger and thumb until you're holding a neat half peanut shell between your thumb and middle finger with the top half of the shell dropping onto the table.

The peanuts inside the shell will be nestled, fully intact and waiting for you to toss them neatly into your mouth.

As the evening lengthens, all around you people will have unsightly piles of crushed peanut shells in front of them. You however, will have only perfect half-shells beside you.

People will notice. I promise. Be prepared to respond to their "how" questions smile. I answer with one word,

"Finesse."

COOKING

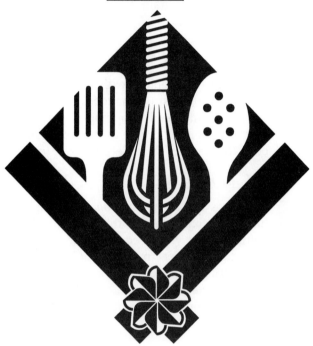

I preface this section with the caveat that I am *not* a gourmet. I'm a *Stone Soup* cook. While I'm not culinarily accomplished, I have found many of the pitfalls presented by even survival level one-handed cooking.

Even if you only eat to live, only cooking to stay alive, these ideas will give you what you need to prepare food despite the two-handedness of this world. If you're a gourmet, what I describe here gives you the building blocks to get you back to messing up your kitchen single-handedly. If cooking and preparing food have been important to you, it'll be upward from here!

Cutting and Slicing

Part of the problem with cutting food, when cooking single-handedly, is that sawing slicing, and chopping require an *other hand,* or some way to *hold* what you cut. Not to worry. You need this one tool:

Cutting Board

This is the an *absolute must* for single-handedly managing in the kitchen. The cutting board you need is modified with two stainless steel nails protruding from the cutting surface tips *"up"* 2½ to 3 inches (*pictured left*), with a rubber-coated bottom or with suction cup *"feet."*

* * * * *

To use your cutting board, simply impale on the nails whatever you want to cut, take your knife, and slice, saw, or chop. The nails hold what you're cutting to the board. The rubber bottom or *suction cups* hold the cutting board to the counter.

You may find, as I have, a rubber-coated bottom version is preferable to the *suction cups:* While the *suction cups* hold the cutting board more firmly to the counter, the cups are more difficult to *unsuction* when it's time to move the cutting board—to rinse it, for example. Suction cups require quite a pull to *unsuction*, and tugging hard at the cutting board inevitably means the juices—from whatever you've just cut—splatter all over when *"pop,"* the *suction cups* do let go.

You'll find a *kazillion* ways to use your cutting board, bagels, unsliced bread, grapefruit, melon, vegetables, preparing chicken or meat, even to help with grating. The following ideas and instructions will get you started.

Bagels

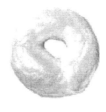

Except for the frozen, *pre-sliced* supermarket bagel *facsimiles*, you may have thought that unless someone else cut them for you, bagels had become only a fond memory from your *two-handed days*.

Au Contraire!

Impale your bagel on the cutting board, vertically. If it's a somewhat oblong bagel, put one of the longer flatter edges along the cutting board.

Turn the cutting board so the bagel is in relief to you (*so you're looking at the bagel as an "I" rather than as an "O"*) Drive a serrated steak knife into the bagel from the top and push the blade all the way through. Still holding the knife handle in the palm of your hand, press your index finger against the top of the bagel, to help with leverage.

Saw the knife blade into the bagel with the heel of your hand, pulling the blade back out by pressing your index finger into the bagel.

Fairly quickly, you'll have cut through half the bagel—the vertical side closest to you. Turn the cutting board 180° and repeat the instructions, above until your bagel is halved. Now, enjoy! If you like, spread on cream cheese, lox, jelly, or butter. *For help with that, see pages 94-95.*

Grapefruit

Impale the grapefruit on your cutting board nails and cut across the fruit sections. Then impale each half skin down, fruit-side up and cut each fruit section away from the section membranes, and then around the perimeter of the skin.

Oranges

See page 101 for a discussion of preparing oranges to eat with one hand.

Knives

Meat Cleaver

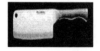

Just because Butchers only use this knife on a block to vigorously separate cuts of meat, doesn't mean that's the only function meat cleavers have in life. Taking an ordinary item and adapting by applying it to not ordinary uses is part of the art of learning to manage single-handedly.

You can use a sharp meat cleaver to pressure cut through flat foods, like Syrian bread, luncheon meats, sliced cheese, Syrian bread pizzas, etc., the types of food which tear when subjected to the back and forth pulling single-handed cutting entails The deep blade and extended handle give you the leverage you need to cut cleanly.

A meat cleaver also helps slice lettuce and cabbage, and half cobs of corn, for example. Your meat cleaver will be coming out of the drawer far more frequently than you ever imagined, especially now that you know to use it for more than simply heavy duty meat cleaving.

Roller knife

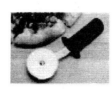

Looking just like a pizza cutter with a stronger, more ergonomic handle, and a sturdier sharper blade, a Roller Knife, in combination with your cutting board easily slices thin breads, the crusts from sliced bread, softer vegetables and fruits, etc. While a Roller Knife won't take care of *all* your cutting needs, it can play an important role in your kitchen.

Knife sharpener

While knives can be sharpened by placing a whetting stone on the counter and drawing the knife blade across, you may have found that unless the stone is a sizable block, it slides on the table, marring your sharpening job.

Try mounting a small knife sharpener on the wall in your kitchen. This way, all you need to do is draw the blade through the sharpener, making knife sharpening a one-handed task. *You can find wall-mountable knife sharpeners at just about any kitchen gadget store or department.*

Grating

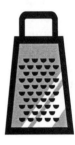

While your food processor does a fine job grating carrots and cheese, you don't always have to take it out just because you're single-handed. Especially when a plain old grater will do the job just as fast and is easier to clean up.

Lay your four-sided grater on your cutting board. Anchor it there by hanging the handle over the nails. If the rubber bottom on your cutting board won't hold to the counter firmly enough. Line up the edge of the cutting board with the edge of the counter so that by standing close to the counter you can brace the cutting board and grater against your abdomen [the first secret: *Body Positioning*].

Because only one end of the grater is braced with your body, you'll only be able to swipe what you're grating across the grater by pulling it toward you. Still, one firm pass across a grater will shred much of an average carrot.

When you're done, the gratings remain inside the grater. Carry the gratings inside the grater over to your mixing bowl and knock the grater against your mixing bowl (*or saucepan*) side so the gratings drop inside for mixing/cooking.

Stirring & Mixing

You've faced the problem—when you don't have an *other* hand to hold the bowl still, the stirring just makes the pan spin around—accomplishing nothing. You can deal with this.

While cooking on the Stove

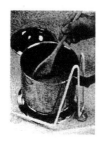

The **Pan Holder** is designed to resolve spinning saucepan syndrome. It fastens to the stove top with rubber suction cups. Between the "*wire folds*" trap the saucepan handle, to hold the pan steady as you stir.

* * * * *

Alternatively, you can try using **Body Positioning** to address this problem. Set the saucepan on one of the front burners so the handle hangs out over the edge of the stove, just enough to catch it with your torso as you stir.

If you choose to use body positioning, *be sure that after you've finished mixing, you twist the handle of the pan around, toward the center of the stove.* Don't leave the handle hanging over the edge. After all that work, you don't want to bump the handle and knock your gourmet culinary creation off the stove and onto the floor—or worse yet onto you.

In a bowl on a Counter

Saucepans:

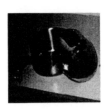

Using a *saucepan* on the counter, with its handle hanging over the edge, and trapped by your abdomen is the simplest way to mix ingredients even when they won't be cooked on the stove—but especially if those ingredients are to be cooked after the mixing.

"Little Octopus / Suction Cup Pads"

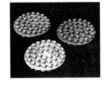

These are indispensable gadgets to which you'll find you resort for countless purposes not *always* cooking related.

Suction cup pads work best when first dampened with water. The water causes them to adhere more tightly against the countertop and to the bottom of your bowl. Lay the dampened pad on the counter. Since you'll be attaching your mixing bowl to the pad, place the pad relatively close to the counter edge, or where ever it's most comfortable for you to work. Firmly press your flat-bottomed mixing bowl onto the suction cup pad. The mixing bowl will stick to the pad which you've stuck to the counter. The suction pad will hold your mixing bowl firmly enough, to stir whatever you're working with, just about as vigorously as you care to stir.

Hand-Held Mixer

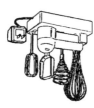

If you do a lot of baking and cooking, too much single-handed mixing and stirring will strain your one wrist—something you want to avoid at all costs! Try a lightweight rechargeable hand-held mixer. Adding this piece of equipment to your kitchen is more expensive than a spoon, and rubber suction pad, but if you like to cook, treat yourself. It's easy to manage single-handedly, and because it can be mounted on a wall bracket next to an outlet, it's always readily accessible.

You can damage your one hand trying to do something like whip egg whites to stiff peaks using only a whisk, single-handedly. Without an _other hand_ to alternate with, your one wrist will ache for days, trust me. This appliance makes an excellent present for the single-handed chef, even if you cook only for yourself.

Food Processor

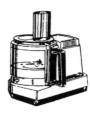

Another _must-have_ for the single-handed cook's kitchen is a food processor. With prices for household electronics and appliances tending steadily downward, you _can_ find a model to suit both your needs and your pocketbook. Be sure to select a model that you can easily assemble and disassemble—one without too many removable pieces that will need to be handled for washing. And, unless your kitchen is large enough to store your food processor on the counter, be sure you can single-handedly move it from where ever you'll store it, to the counter.

To use your food processor, measure dry goods and liquids, and with help from your cutting board (see *page 120),* cut ingredients to a size your food processor can accommodate. Adjust the cutting blades or fittings as directed in the manufacturer's instructions, then fill up the food processor bowl and let the appliance do its thing. *What could be better?*

Opening

Getting into stuff, is a consideration for onee-handed cook. Today, ingredients come in packaging designed to protect in transit. So carefully are products packaged that even two-handed folks have trouble.

Box tops

Baking soda, breakfast cereals, rice, and even laundry detergent boxes are designed with a perforated semi-circle you're supposed to push your thumb into. How do you do that, without holding the box steady with an *other hand?*

Lay the box on the narrow side opposite the perforated semi-circle for your thumb to push into. Gravity should allow you to press your thumb firmly enough to break the perforations and pierce the box.

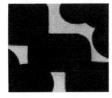

You may find a Dycem sheet (*pictured left*) under the box adds stability.

* * * * *

If the narrow edge is so narrow the box doesn't feel stable enough, try using the First Secret, *Body Positioning*. Step closer to the counter so you can brace the box between the counter edge and your torso. You'll have more room to maneuver your one hand, if you lay the box crosswise to the counter—so the bottom of the box rests against your torso. Also, pressing against the perforated semi-circle with your thumb will press the box into your body (*chest, abdomen, or thigh depending on your height and the height of your counter*).

* * * * *

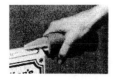

Alternatively, if neither procedure works for you, you, because you're working with your non-dominant hand or don't have the dexterity or strength in your one hand, can try a *box top opener*. It's a handy gadget designed to break through the perforated semi-circle and when lifted, tearing away the box top. *Talk with your Occupational Therapist (OT) about a box top opener.*

Cans

Don't even think about using that hand crank can opener still taking up space in your kitchen drawer. Put it out in the next garage sale. Or if your *other* hand might heal, pack it away in the attic until after the healing.

Can Openers

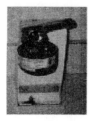

Many electric can opener models can be managed single-handedly. Beware though, models vary, so you'll need test before you buy. When you go shopping for your electric can opener, bring a can with you. Even if the floor samples aren't plugged in, and they probably won't be, you'll still be able determine whether a particular model will work for you.

To use your electric can opener, hold the can between your thumb, and middle ring, and pinkie fingers. Place your thumb and middle finger close to the rim of the can. *Leave your index finger free.*

With the can opener handle half way open, slip the can under the magnet so the blade is lined up to pierce the can when the handle is brought down. Reach for the handle with your index finger, hooking that finger over the handle. Bring down the handle just enough for the magnet to catch hold of the can. ***You must choose the a can opener model with a magnet strong enough to hold the can in place without your holding it.***

This is a critical test. If the magnet isn't strong enough to hold the can, this is not the model for you. Test another one.

Once home with your new can opener, you want to actually open a can:

Hold the can, as close to the rim as possible, between your thumb, middle, ring, and pinkie fingers. *Leave your index finger free.* With the can opener handle open half way, slip the can under the magnet so the blade is lined up to pierce the can when the handle is brought down.

Reach for the handle with your index finger and bring down the handle just enough for the magnet to catch hold of the can. Let go of the can and take hold of the handle, bring the handle down so the blade pierces the can and the gears clamp onto the can rim. Let go of the can and press down firmly on the handle, opening the can.

* * * * *

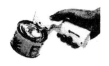

If a counter top can opener doesn't work for you—perhaps you haven't the strength or dexterity you need in your one hand--d*on't despair.* Try a hand-held cordless, rechargeable can opener. Designed to be used with one-hand, this can opener (*pictured left*) pierces the can and *"walks"* around the can top without your needing to add any pressure. Placing a piece of **Dycem** (see *page 129*) on the counter underneath the can will help stabilize the can while using this type of can opener.

Sardine

You don't *have* to use the aluminum peel back key arrangements sardine can manufacturers design into their cans. Sardine cans can be opened far more easily using your electric can opener *(see "Cans" above).*

Frozen juice

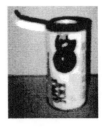

Some frozen orange juice cans are designed to be opened by peeling away a plastic strip. Do this single-handedly by laying the juice container on the counter top. Pinch the loose edge of the plastic strip between your index finger and thumb and rest the palm of your hand and fingers loosely on the juice container. Pull up on the plastic tab. Between gravity and the weight of your hand on the juice container, the plastic tab will pull loose, rolling the juice container under your hand.

After you've pulled off the plastic strip, pop off the metal lid. Now wrap your hand around the juice container and turn it up-side-down over a wide necked pitcher or your blender. If you lightly squeeze the cardboard container, between the squeezing and the warmth of your hand, the concentrate will drop out of the container and into the pitcher.

The easiest and, in my opinion, most delicious way to make juice from frozen concentrate is in the blender. Drop the concentrate into the blender, add the appropriate measures of water, put on the blender lid, and switch on the blender to break up the concentrate mixing it with the water. When done, you'll have a delicious, frothy juice drink. You may never drink your juices any other way.

Jars

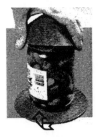

Dycem mat

First tap the lid on the floor, this seems to help loosen the vacuum seal. Place the jar high up between your thighs, a couple of inches below your crotch. As you press your thighs together, to hold onto the jar or bottle, your adductor muscles will grip the jar and hold it tight. With your one hand, twist off the cover. Using this technique, I've been known to open jars no one else could budge...

Reversing this procedure (*without the tapping part of course* ☺) enables you to securely close a jar.

To help you better grip the lid, you can use a rubber jar opener mat. After settling the jar high up between your thighs, pick up the jar-opener mat so it covers the palm of your hand. Now, turn your hand over and grip the jar lid with the jar-opener mat between the palm of your hand and the lid. The mat will hang over the sides of the lid. Twist the cover.

Likewise, reversing the above, enables you to securely close a jar.

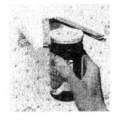

Alternatively, you can install an under-counter or cabinet *jar lid opener/tightener*. It consists of a hardened steel knurled "V" shaped gripper. Tap the lid on a threshold or against your wooden cutting board. Then, holding the jar, slide the lid into the "V" as far as it will go. When the lid is gripped in the "V," twist the jar counter-clockwise to open and clockwise to close. (*see Resources, page 246 to find this gadget.*)

Milk Cartons & Jugs

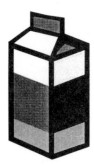

Whenever possible, select milk cartons with a *built-in* plastic spout over the creased cardboard opening. Not only does the plastic spout pour more easily, but it's easier to open. *Do be careful about container size. When two-handed people pour from a gallon jug, they have that "other hand" to help support the weight.*

Ice Trays

Most ice trays are designed to be turned upside-down over the ice bucket and then bent in an arc or twisted between *two* hands to dislodge the cubes. This simply doesn't work single-handedly.

Fortunately, the folks at Rubbermaid® have manufactured a flexible ice tray that empties when simply turned up-side-down. Just hold it up-side-down over your ice bucket!

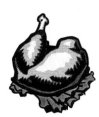

Special Tricks

Chicken

If you eat chicken, and you're also watching your cholesterol intake, you'll want be able to remove the skin and fat before cooking. Here's how:

You could buy already skinned chicken, but why? Just because you're one-handed? Buying chicken that way is more expensive, so do it yourself this way:

Before starting, gather:
- a sharp ***Scissors***,
- your <u>Cutting Board</u>
- a ***Large Jar*** with a wide opening (*a 2½ pound peanut butter jar is perfect—glass is better because the weight adds stability*), and a ***Plastic Bag***. (*reusing old bread bags recycles.*)

You'll want to set yourself up near the sink since your one hand gets all *ooey*, and *gooey* working with chicken. Working close to the sink allows you to more easily rinse your hand as you need.

Line the inside of the jar with the plastic bag, rolling the edge of the bag down the sides of the jar. As you peel and cut the skin and fat away from the chicken, drop that into your bag-lined jar. The jar allows you to single-handedly discard chicken debris in the bag for *odor-free* until trash day.

Now for the chicken. Place your cutting board on the counter so the nails are farthest from the edge of the counter and the opposite end of the board hangs an inch or so over the counter edge. Impale a piece of chicken, skin side up, on the cutting board nails. (*I prefer leg and thigh sections—the dark meat—but have found this procedure works equally as well with breast or back pieces.*

Stand with your body close enough to the counter that the edge of the cutting board rests against your abdomen. This provides the leverage you'll need to tear the skin away from the meat.

Pick at the edge of the chicken piece that's farthest from you, and work the fingers of your one hand between the skin and meat. Keep picking at the skin, as if you're scratching an itch, until you raise a flap of skin.

Grab hold of that flap between your index finger and thumb, or however you can, and pull it toward you, along the nails. If the cutting board weren't wedged against your abdomen, it would slide across the counter as you pull at the chicken skin.

Use your scissors to clip tough fibers of myelin sheath you can't tear away. Between pulling to tear the skin away, and clipping with the scissors, the skin will separate from the meat. As you cut, drop the skin in your plastic bag-lined jar and then cut away the now-exposed *globulars* of fat with your scissors. It's messy work, no matter how many hands you use. But it *can* be done single-handedly...

Garlic

Garlic has been promoted recently as the panacea for all our ills including cold or flu, and even broken hearts. Whether or not any of it's true, garlic is a great seasoning and is frequently called for, so you might as well know how to handle it easily with one hand.

You may have thought peeling the tough outer shell-like skin from cloves of fresh garlic wasn't possible to manage single-handedly, unless you pierced the shell with your thumb nail digging into the garlic meat. Of course that way, the garlic juice burns the soft skin under your nail and, no matter how vigorously you wash after each encounter you smell like garlic, for days.

New!

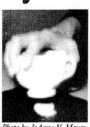

Photo by JoAnne N. Mayer

There is an easier way. Break cloves away from the garlic head and lay the half moon-shaped cloves on the counter so they would rock if you pressed on one tip.

Holding a teacup, with the palm of your hand covering the rim. Bang the bottom of the teacup down onto each garlic clove one at a time. The impact of the teacup bottom on the garlic clove cracks the hard clove shell so you can easily peel it away, and release the garlic meat.

If you use a wooden cutting board, consider chopping your garlic on a glass saucer rather than on your cutting board so the garlic juices won't seep into the wood grains of your cutting board.

Garlic is great, but mixed with the oranges, apples, and the many other uses you have for your cutting board... Use the teacup groove in a saucer as a ridge against which you can trap the garlic clove allowing you to cut the clove in half. Then turn the clove halves onto the flat cut and chop finely as you need.

Cracking Eggs

Secure your mixing bowl to the counter with a suction cup pad (see *page126)*. Hold the egg cupped in the palm of your one hand. Firmly and squarely rap the egg on the rum of the mixing bowl opening the eggshell with a gash the width of the mixing bowl rim. Holding the egg over the mixing bowl, work your thumb and ring finger into that gash, prying the crack open and releasing the yolk and albumen (*egg white*) into the mixing bowl. I'm told this is how cordon bleu chefs crack eggs, in the world's finest kitchens.

CLEANING UP

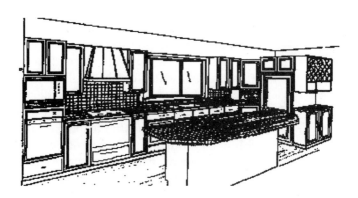

Rule #1 is *"Keep ahead of it."* Don't let utensils, pots, pans, and dishes pile up while you cook. All the while you're working in the kitchen, rinse and wash pots, pans, and utensils as you use them. Place those going in the dishwasher into the dishwasher and put away ingredients. As long as you don't allow the kitchen to get ahead of you, you'll be able to handle your kitchen messes single-handedly.

The other reason to keep up with the mess while you cook is that to cook effectively single-handedly, you need clear counter space where you can put your project down while you work with it.

Rule #2 is *"Keep it Handy."* If you're at all like me, you'll more likely follow Rule #1 if all the tools and ingredients you need for the project you're working on are close at hand.

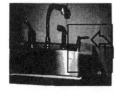

Soap Dispenser

Most stainless steel kitchen sinks are designed so features such as a water filter, a sprayer, or **Soap Dispenser** can be added as desired. A built-in soap dispenser (*pictured left*) which can be easily added to your kitchen is a *must-have* in the one-handed kitchen. You'll use it every day. And just you watch, after helping clean up following your next party, half your two-handed friends will be adding soap dispensers to their kitchens. My mom did. *Trend setting is such fun.*

Just think, with a soap dispenser, as you single-handedly wash dishes, you no longer need pick up the dish washing liquid bottle to squirt soap onto your sponge. Secondly, mounted to your sink, your soap dispenser won't tip over in the under sink cabinet, and it's simple to refill!

Dish towel Holder

Most kitchens are laid out with dishtowels stashed in drawers. Why? It only means that with your hand dripping wet, you have to open a drawer to take out a dish towel whenever you need one. What a disincentive to washing your one hand while working in the kitchen...

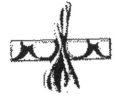

Try mounting a plastic **Dish-Towel Holder** (*see left*) on your refrigerator door, a central location in the kitchen, fairly close to the sink. Where better to hang a decorative kitchen towel, or two, or three?

Sponges

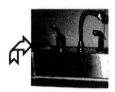

One _"Keep it Handy"_ trick is to keep a damp, lightly soaped sponge on the stainless steel ledge between the faucet and knobs, ready where you'll need it. That way, you won't have to open the cabinet under the sink, fish around for the sponge, then push the cabinet door closed before you can wipe up the whatever.

Faucets

If you're making decisions on the whole kitchen design, including faucets, why not select a single control for both hot and cold water. Regulating water temperature single-handedly is vastly easier when there's only one control to contend with.

Cabinets

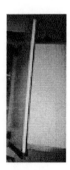

Again, if you're re-doing your kitchen, or starting from scratch, you'll find that choosing cabinet doors and drawers that open by pulling on a beveled groove along the bottom of the wall cabinet doors and top of the floor cabinet doors and drawers, rather than with knobs, are easier when managing a kitchen single-handedly.

If the doors and drawers open with a beveled groove, you can be holding the glass, plate, or whatever you want to put inside, and still open the cabinet door or drawer even if only the tip of your one pinkie finger is the sole digit available to open the door or drawer.

Countertops and tables

You *could* just wipe crumbs and scraps off the counter or table onto the floor, and then sweep the floor. But as you'll see, *one-handed sweeping. (Turn to page 167 for ideas on sweeping)*, isn't all that much easier.

Instead, furnish your kitchen with a rectangular 13-gallon plastic trash receptacle. Even mostly full, you can maneuver this size container single-handedly.

When you wipe the counter or table, work the scraps and crumbs into a pile near the edge of the counter. Move your kitchen trash receptacle, in line with the pile and wedge the trash bucket between your body and the floor cabinets with one of the longer sides of the trash bucket just below the counter overhang and flat against the floor cabinets below the counter. Now, wipe the scraps and crumbs into the trash receptacle.

If there aren't floor cabinets under your counter, or if you're sponging a table top, wipe the scraps and crumbs into a pile a few inches from the edge of the table. Move your trash receptacle, into position, under the table and across from the pile of scraps and crumbs, but sticking out from under the table/counter enough to catch the debris when you wipe the scraps and crumbs into the trash receptacle.

Dishes, & Platters

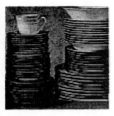

Just like two-handed dishwashers, you still want to rinse off your plates, before stacking them in the sink. Rinsing makes the scrubbing doable.

Prepare a Sponge by dampening it with hot water. Squirt a few drops of dish washing liquid onto the center of the sponge. And squeeze it, evenly distributing the soap and working-up suds.

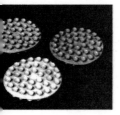

Dampen a _Suction cup pad "Little Octopus" (see left)_ with water. Then lay it on the floor of the sink. If you're working in a sink with corners, position the pad three to four inches out from one of the _near_ corners (_one of the corners closest to you, as opposed to the **far** corners closer to the kitchen back wall_) and two to three inches from the side. That way, you can use the walls of the sink to leverage against vigorous scrubbing. With little suction cups on both sides of the suction cup pad, the pad sticks both to the floor of the sink and to the underside of the plate you intend to wash, effectively working with you like an _other_ hand.

Scrub the inside of the plate. The suction cups hold the plate quite tightly allowing you to scrub forcefully. Lift up the plate and rinse it. To wash the bottom, turn over the plate, resting the rim over the suction pad. Most likely, there won't be a surface flat enough for the suction cups to grip on, but if you've rinsed the plates, the bottoms don't need to be scrubbed, just wiped a few times with a sudsy sponge. Resting the plate against a couple of rubber suction pads gives you just enough friction to accomplish that.

But if food on the back of the plate needs *elbow grease* attention, you'll want to reposition the plate by sticking the suction pad a couple of inches from the *far* corner opposite the hand you use. This way. With the edge of the plate nestled among the suction cups, it is also wedged against both the back and side walls of the sink. Between the suction cup pad, the back and the side of the sink, you should have the plate settled firmly enough to scrub the underside clean. Continue scrubbing as necessary and rinse.

Flatware

Prepare your Sponge as described above (see *page143*). Lay your prepared sponge on the flat ledge beside the faucet with the edge of the sponge in line with the inside edge of the sink.

Knives

First rinse the blade. Then, holding the knife by its handle, wipe the blade, across your sudsy sponge. Push down on the blade, bending it lightly—Pressure increases the friction, helping to clean off the food residue. Flip the knife over and wipe the other side of the blade against the sudsy sponge. Keep wiping both sides until the knife is clean, then rinse.

Forks

Wash forks similarly to *knives* (*above*) by firmly wiping the prongs of each fork across your sudsy sponge. Forks won't bend like a knife blade, so you need to use the angle you wipe at to increase pressure on the prongs wiping across the sponge. Turn the fork back to front and wipe until it's clean, and rinse.

Spoons

When wiping the outside of each spoon bowl across the sponge, you'll find it cleans more effectively to swing the spoon handle back and forth as you wipe. To clean inside the spoon bowl, wipe the spoon across the one corner of the sponge filling the bowl with sudsy sponge. As with knives and forks above, keep wiping until the spoon is clean, then rinse.

Serving Utensils

You'll use the same basic procedures as described above for washing flatware, to wash serving knives and forks. When dealing with **serving spoons**, however, it's easier to rest the butt end of the handle on the floor of the sink and pick up your sudsy sponge, washing the bowl of the spoon by folding the sponge over the bowl between your thumb and middle finger.

Using the sink floor for leverage, pinch the serving spoon bowl between your thumb and middle and ring fingers, with your thumb pressing the sponge into the bowl of the spoon, massage both sides of the spoon bowl between your thumb and fingers. Continue massaging until the serving spoon is clean, and then rinse.

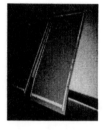

plastic place mats

Line your place mats side-by-side on the counter perpendicular to the counter edge with about three inches overhanging the counter edge.

Unless you're wearing an apron or *"work"* clothes, the overhanging three inches should be the *least* dirty, or sticky. Use an ammonia based cleaning solution in a spray-bottle. Lightly dampen your sponge, then spray a fine coat of cleaning solution onto each place mat, but not on the three inches you've left hanging over the edge. Let the spray soak in a moment or so.

Lean against the counter, trapping those three inches of overhanging now clean place mat between your body and the counter. By trapping the place mat like this, you'll be able to briskly scrub with your sponge, and get the place mat really clean. Scrub at the stains that didn't lift off easily. Then, rinse the sponge and wipe off the dampness and spray cleaner.

To finish up, step back from the counter and rotate the place mat 180° so the three inches that were trapped between your body and the counter are lying on the counter now and the now clean *other* end hangs over the edge.

Press your body into the counter to trap the *new* three inches of place mat hanging over the edge between your body and counter. Spray the still dirty 3" strip of place mat, and wipe. One done. Three? Five? to go...

Pots & Pans

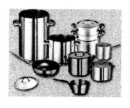

You may not want to take a job washing pots and pans in a restaurant—but then again, with these tips and ideas, maybe you will. In any case, there's no need to let the pots and pans pile up in the sink until you prevail upon good-natured two-handed friends and neighbors to help you.

Save those good-natured people for occasions when help is absolutely necessary—when you need a huge steamer trunk in the attic moved downstairs...

Start by soaking everything with any left over food residue especially baked-on or burned-in. Two-handers do, why not you?

Prepare your sponge as described in *__Flatware__* *(page 144)* and set up a suction cup pad see page 126, "*__Little Octopus__*" laying it on the floor of the sink.

If you're working on a pan with a handle and in a sink with corners, it's helpful to position the pad so the pot is wedged into one of the *near* corner (*the corner closest to you and the hand you use, as opposed to one of the far corners closer to the kitchen wall*) opposite from the hand you use. That way, the sides of the sink add leverage if the scrubbing needs to be vigorous. Because suction cup pads have suction cups on both sides, they stick to the floor of the sink and the underside of the pot you're washing and effectively work for you, just like an *other* hand.

Pan Scraper

This clever little plastic tool enables you to scrape away the oatmeal that cooked too long this morning, or got left in the pot after you ate, while you showered and dressed—the morning routine. With a pan scraper you can deal with the five-alarm chili, the goulash, the stew, the whatever that "*caught*" and stuck to the bottom of the pan. My pan scraper was an *impulse buy* I noticed by the cash register at the local True Value Hardware and Housewares store.

All you do is soak the stuck food stuff and then stick the pan to the floor of the sink with a *suction cup pad (see page126)*. With the pan firmly stuck to your suction cup pad, wedged into the *near* corner opposite the hand you use, and the pot's handle against the side of the sink to keep the pan from twisting out of the suction cup pad's grip while you work at it, hold the scraper between your thumb and index finger like a guitar pick. Fit one of the curved corners (*each corner is a different arc to better scrape different volume pans*) to the inside curve of your saucepan and scrape the pan scraper around the circumference, lifting off stuck on food.

Leftover Food Storage

Effectively storing your leftovers not only keeps food tasting fresh, but also the refrigerator smelling fresh, and helps prevent messy refrigerator spills.

There are plenty of containers designed to store leftovers. Some are better than others. Single-handers want to **avoid the round heavy plastic containers in a variety of sizes, with the beige lids**. These containers are terrific for *two-handed* people. They seal tightly, go into the dishwasher, and are *microwaveable*. But single-handedly, it's hard to remove the covers—*so why bother?* Give away any you already have in your kitchen, and **don't** buy these, otherwise you'll be saving leftovers in your refrigerator you can't get into easily, and what's the point?

If you've already been through trying to get into the *just-enough for lunch* leftovers from the night before, that your friend so carefully tucked away in a plastic bag sealed with a *twist-tie* turned again and again, you know some of the issues. Let's resolve them.

plastic containers

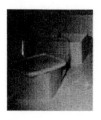

The best plastic containers for one-handed food storage also happen to be the most easily stored and least expensive. The square one- and two-pint containers which are typically shrink-wrapped in packages of four and eight. These work best because the covers are easy to put on and remove, they're lightweight, and they stack, for easy storage.

plastic bags

Instead of plastic wrap which is hard to manage single-handedly, use plastic bags. One way to easily get food into the plastic bag is to slide the platter of leftovers right into the mouth of plastic bag. This way, the platter weighs-down the plastic bag and you can push the leftover food off the platter into the bag.

* * * * *

Alternatively, line a glass container with a plastic bag, described in *"**Dealing with Chicken**," on page 135.*

Closures

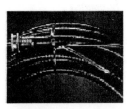

Twist ties are a beast to twist closed single-handedly and as bad if not worse to untwist open. Don't bother. *Throw away every twist tie in your kitchen.* That way, friends helping out after dinner won't be tempted to use them.

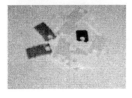

Plastic Tabs used to close bags of bakery goods like bread, rolls, and bagels, easily managed with one hand, are a one-handers' dream. Keep a stash readily available somewhere in your kitchen.

To use a Plastic Tab, once the bag is filled, grab the bag at the opening end between the palm of your hand and your middle, ring and pinkie fingers. Lift the bag so it isn't touching the counter.

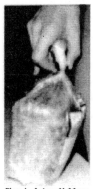

Photo by JoAnne N. Mayer

Twist the opening end of the bag closed. Press against the filled part of the bag with your thumb and index finger, starting the filled part spinning so the "neck" twists to a smaller diameter.

When the "neck" of the bag has twisted small enough to slide the plastic tab over, lower the bag so the bottom rests on the counter to stop the spinning and keep the bag from untwisting. With your thumb and index finger pick up a plastic tabs with the opening away from your fingers. Curl your wrist inward, bringing the tab close to the neck of the bag, and slip the opening over the twisted neck of the bag, clamping the bag shut.

* * * * *

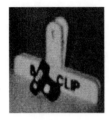

Bag Clips are another option to securely close opened food bags (*particularly opened potato chip bags, cookies, etc.*) **Bag Clips** first appeared in stores jumbo sized, suitable clamping opened snack foods bags but are now available in medium and small sizes, so you can match a clip to need.

* * * * *

Using a **Bag Clip** is fairly straight forward. Shake the contents of the bag to the bottom, lie the large, stiffer bags (*for example, a potato chip bag*) on the counter. Smooth the open end and fold it once or twice. After you've finished folding, with your middle finger pressed down on one corner of the folded-closed opening, scrape your thumbnail down the folded edge, *"inch-worming"* your thumb nail and middle finger, down the length of the fold so the crease is pressed firm. This way, the fold will stay put when you move your hand to pick up the bag clip. Slide the bottom of the bag to the edge of the counter and step close enough to the counter that the bottom of the bag rests against your abdomen taking advantage of that first secret, *Body Positioning, introduced on page 11).*

Pick up the bag clip, squeezing the handles between your fingers and the palm of your hand. Slide the opened clip over the folded edge of the bag. With your body positioned to trap the bag, you can release the bag clip so it firmly clamps the whole bag preserving the contents.

To *bag clip* a plastic bag closed, once the bag is filled, twist the opening of the bag as described above (see *page151)*.

When the *neck* of the bag has twisted small enough to be clamped by a small bag clip, rest the bottom if the bag on the counter, to stop the spinning and keep the *neck* from untwisting. With your thumb and index finger pick up the bag clip. Squeezing the clip handles between your index finger and thumb, open the clip. Curl your wrist inward, bringing the bag clip close to the neck of the bag. Loosen your hold on the bag clip levers so the clip clamps over the *neck* of the bag.

Marking frozen leftovers

You'll want to label all those plastic containers and bags of leftovers stashed in your freezer. Two-handers use masking tape and an indelible marker, but unless you can find a masking-tape tape dispenser, masking tape is hard to manage single-handedly.

Try using *file folder labels*. Mark the label in pencil, peel it off the non-stick backing, and press it against the plastic container you want to label—next time you use the container, erase & re-label... This way, even one-handedly, you'll have a well organized freezer.

HOUSEHOLD CHORES

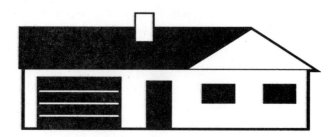

Laundry

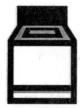

It's one of those necessary evils that goes with independent living, something we all must deal with. To top it off, laundry never gets *done*! Shortly after the clothes finish tumbling in the drier, you realize what you were wearing is soiled and so into the hamper go those clothes, ready for the next wash.

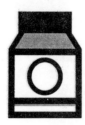

Emptying the Dryer: The best gadget to help accomplish this task, is a large binder clip (*pictured left*). I keep mine in the laundry room—but if you take your laundry to the Laundromat, keep your binder clip with your laundry detergent, fabric softener, and dryer sheets.

When you're ready to remove your clean dry clothes from the dryer, open the dryer door and fish out your laundry bag. Clip the laundry bag to the dryer door so the bag opening is stretched between the top corners of the dryer door. The *not hinged* corner will catch enough of the bag to hold it firm. Clip your binder clip over the bag and the *hinged* dryer door corner. Now with your one hand, you can easily stuff your clothes into the bag.

Bed Sheet Storage

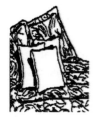

You don't have to struggle with carefully folding sheets to stack in the linen closet. Nobody does that any more. A November 1993 back page _Time Magazine_ essay explained "*in the 90s we no longer have to devote endless time and energy to homemaking and housework. We're just too busy.*"

* * * * *

But if you want to show yourself bed sheets can be neatly folded single-handedly... Go for it. Here's how.

Lay out the top sheet over a freshly made bed. Painstakingly bring the corners from the foot of the bed up to those at the head of the bed, one after the other. Then straighten out the fold by lightly pulling each fold-corner down over the edge of the bed toward the floor. Just a light tug, and then back toward the foot of the bed a little, maybe an inch or so.

Then, one at a time, bring the *fold-*corners up to meet the corners at the head of the bed. Straighten the double fold the same way, by lightly pulling each *fold-*corner first down over the edge of the bed toward the floor a bit, just a light tug, and then back toward the foot of the bed a little, just an inch or so. Keep bringing the *fold* corners up to meet the corners at the head of the bed until you've folded the sheet as narrowly as you need to fit on your linen closet shelf.

Now pick up one of the bottom side corners and lay it on the sheet section on the far side of the bed, but not hanging over the edge, not yet. You want to be careful gravity doesn't bring the whole thing down to the floor, in which case you'd have to start all over again...

Slip your arm through this new fold. Drag the sheet, now folded into a strip, up so the other two side corners are drawn onto the bed: Now that the sheet is down to a *single-handleable* size, you can easily finish folding to fit the closet space.

* * * * *

Fitted sheets are foldable too.

Lay-out a clean fitted sheet atop your freshly made bed. Make the corners at the head of the bed neat by folding the sides (*the four inches of material that make the sheet fit*) over onto the flat of the sheet and then, repeat the process you just used for the flat sheet.

Sure, you can do all this folding, but why bother? Fold your sheets once, only to prove to yourself you can—not that you're going to every week.

Instead, lighten up, Mom will never know. An alternative to folding is to dig the pillow case out of the dryer and clip it to the dryer door with a binder clip, the way you did your laundry bag (see *above, page 154)*. Stuff the other pillowcase, and matching flat, and fitted sheets inside the binder clipped pillowcase.

Pack your pillowcase stuffed with sheets into the linen closet until you need those sheets to make a bed, no more rummaging around to find matching sheets minutes before company arrives! The fitted sheet will stretch smooth. The top sheet will flatten after you tuck it in, and under the weight of the blanket and spread. *No one will ever figure your secret!*

Pairing socks.

Don't you despise wasting time rummaging through a drawer searching for a matched pair of socks? The only solution is to pair socks together as they come out of the dryer or as they go into the drawer.

Single-handedly, it's automatic to use your teeth to help fold the cuff of one sock over the other. I did it that way, until I worked out this next trick.

* * * * *

First time, try this with a thickly cuffed pair of ankle socks.

Lay the other of the pair on top of it's mate, matching the socks cuff-to-cuff, heel-to-heel, toe-to-toe. Pinch the pair together between your thumb and fingers by sliding your thumb into the opening of the bottom sock and by loosely straddling your four fingers over the cuff of the top sock. With your hands holding both socks as described, pick up the socks. Firmly rub the loose bottom sock <u>cuff</u> up your thigh, pressing your fingertips against your thigh driving them inside the folds of the material. Now roll your wrist over. Use your thumb to coax the bottom sock cuff over the top sock.

Fitted Sheets

Before I came up with this trick, I suffered many a night restlessly trying to get a night's sleep after the corners of my fitted sheet had pulled away from the mattress. I was stuck with a long uncomfortable night lying on a lumped together bottom sheet and mattress pad.

These days, my fitted bottom sheet fits as snugly as my two-handed mother's, and it doesn't take any longer to get it that way. You too can securely fit bottom sheets onto the corners of your mattresses.

Lay the bottom sheet, arranged so the four corners line up with the correct mattress corners. (*Don't skip this step. Inevitably you'll be halfway through only to find, you've fitted side corners to the headboard corners, and have to start again...*) Let the fitted corners of the sheets fold back forming a pocket with the inside seam exposed.

The first corner is the most difficult because there's nothing to leverage against. It's easiest to start with the headboard corner on the side of the arm you use. (_If you use your right arm, then start with the headboard right corner. If you use your left arm, start with the headboard left corner_). Lift that mattress corner with your one hand and slide a knee underneath.(_I use the knee of the leg on the same side as the arm I use._)

With your hand resting flat against the mattress and your fingers outstretched, slip your hand into the _pocket_ formed by the fitted sheet corner. Your fingers should be in the fitted sheet corner point with the gathered elastic resting on the top of your hand (_not your palm_).

Slide your hand and the fitted sheet corner toward the mattress corner resting on your knee. When the pad of your middle finger reaches the mattress corner, just before it goes over the edge, arch your wrist. _This forces the elastic to "roll" down your hand toward your fingertips._ With your fingers, work the elastic over the mattress corner, and down under.

Proceed to the next mattress corner, either the same-side at the footboard, or opposite side at the headboard. The remaining corners are easier due to the tension from each corner already fitted to the mattress, For the third and fourth corners, you probably won't find it necessary to lift the mattress corner up onto your knee—only the first and perhaps the second corners.

Hanging clothes

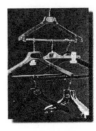

The easiest way to put **blouses and jackets** onto hangers is to lay the piece of clothing out flat, (*Your bed is the perfect place for this*) with the sleeves out-stretched and one of the front plackets fully brought over the back, the other placket only partially brought over, leaving a space to slip the hanger through. Slide the hanger under the folded-over front placket and into the sleeve, then the other and then pick up the shirt by the hanger, and hang it in your closet.

For **trousers or skirts**, arrange these on your bed with the waistband lined up, front on top of back. You *can* use clip skirt hangers single-handedly, but the easiest way to hang slacks, and skirts are *plastic factory clip hangers* designers and many stores use to display their wares. These smaller, 10" white plastic hangers use a metal "**C**" clip to clamp the waistband of your trousers and skirts onto the hanger.

* * * * *

When you've gone out, and it's cold outside, you'll probably want to hang up your coat. Your host/hostess, will usually be more than happy to deal with your coat for you. Don't struggle with a coat hanger in public. You know you can do it yourself, but it's not worth proving it publicly. While chatting, just slip out of your coat and hand it to whomever greets you.

Hand Sewing

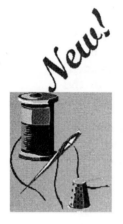

It's going to happen. No question about it. You're going to pop a button, split a seam *"just a little,"* pull down a bit of a hem, or tear a piece of clothing you just have to wear... And that'll happen on the day not a single two-handed someone is anywhere to be found.

Not to worry. Hand sewing single-handedly isn't *easy*, but it is doable.

Choose a well-lighted place with a table beside the chair. A chair with an upholstered arm on the side of the hand you use is preferable. Lacking that, find a footstool and be wearing a pair of loose-fitting long pants.

Gather your needle, thread, scissors, *and if it's a seam or a tear you're sewing* three or four straight pins also. Sit down and cut a length of thread sufficient to do the job at hand—*too much and the thread will inevitably tangle, knotting in just the wrong place.*

Threading the Needle

Stick the tip of your needle just deeply enough in the upholstered chair arm to stand upright by itself. (*If there is no uphol-stered chair arm, use the material of your pant leg—the folds at the inside of your knee. Raise your knee as high as possible, using the foot-stool and stick the needle as vertically as possi-ble into the folds of material.*)

With the needle standing upright draw the freshly cut end of thread through the eye. You may need to rotate the needle so the eye is parallel to your sight-line in or-der to thread the needle. Once threaded, draw the thread through the eye so the ends match up.

As with two-handed sewing, some jobs are more efficiently accomplished with doubled thread. Others finish better when a single strand is used. Buttons, for exam-ple, are probably best affixed to your clothing with the thread doubled whereas a seam, rent, tear, or hem will look better if you use a single thread.

Once that decision is made, it's time to knot your thread. Wet a couple inches of the thread end/s (running the thread across your tongue works for this. *That's the way two-handed seamstresses do it.*

With the needle still stuck into the up-holstered arm of your chair/the material of your pant leg, trap the thread end/s you plan to knot with your thumbnail against the pad of your index finger. By *circling* your index finger, wrap the thread around the tip of your index finger snugly but not tightly. Now by rubbing the pad of your thumb over the thread end/s roll the thread *circle wrapped* around your index fingertip. Two or three rubs and you'll succeed in rubbing the encircled thread off the tip of your finger, tangling the end in the circle. By catching the tangle between your thumb and middle finger nails and gently pulling away from the needle you'll turn that tangle into a knot.

You're now ready to get to the sewing part of this project.

I use my knee *on the same side as the arm I use*, to position the item I'm sewing. When you use a knee, it would be easy to catch the material of your pant leg and sew it together to the shirt cuff, skirt hem, whatever you're sewing. And man, is that a beast that is to rectify...

That's why I recommend wearing shorts when possible (*and using a chair with an upholstered arm*). Otherwise, pull your loose-fitting pant leg up over your knee and out of the way.

The trick to hand sewing single-handedly lies in consciously positioning your project so gravity works with you.

Buttons

Position the shirt placket (*the part of the shirt/blouse where the buttons are affixed*) "*finished side*" up and draped over your knees so the exact place you want to sew the button is suspended between your knees. Lay the button on the placket where it belongs. Take your needle and reaching between your knees press the tip of the needle up into the back side of the placket under one of the holes in the button. Holding the needle between your thumb and middle finger, use your index finger to stabilize the button. Gravity on the placket will allow you to stick the needle into the material and work it through one of the holes in the button enough to grab the needle between your thumb and index or middle finger pad and draw the thread through until the knot at the end of your thread seats against the material. Push the needle through the next hole in the button (*Some people go with the diagonals so the thread makes an "X" in the center of the button. Others go adjacent so the thread pattern on the button is "=" or "□."*)

Me? I try to use a thread color that blends into the button so no one will notice how I sewed it on because coming up from the bottom next time might not fit into the "X" or "=" pattern... Now that you've done the first two stitches, repeat, repeat, and repeat. *To tie off the end of the thread*:   From the top push the needle through a hole in the button at an angle so it doesn't go through the material underneath, from the bottom, push the needle through the material underneath the button but not through one of the holes in the button. Wrap the thread around and around the stitches you've made through the button and material. Leave the last turn loose so you can run the needle through the loop. Now draw the thread tight and cut it.

Hems, Tears, or Rips

These instructions assume you're working on repairs as opposed to hemming a whole skirt or pant leg. For a hemming job, everyone needs someone else to mark and or pin up the hem while you model the garment. I've used the following method to re-sew a three inch section of blue jeans side seam at the thigh, repair a not-seam tear in the collar of my favorite winter jacket, and for dozens of other sewing projects.

With your knees bare (_if you ever pricked a finger of your other hand when sewing two-handedly, be prepared to prick one or both of your knees. It doesn't hurt all that much..._) position the part of clothing to be sewed on the knee corresponding with the hand you use. Use a footstool to raise your knee that much closer to your eyes and one hand.

Work the two sides of the tear together with your fingers, pinning as necessary, or arrange the hem as it should lie and pin to hold it that way. Once you have the area needing stitches pieced together, with that area on the bend of your knee, pinch your knees together catching some of the surrounding material. This adds some stability to the area you'll stitch while you draw the needle in and out.

With everything so organized—*the organizing is the most difficult part*—your only remaining decisions are what stitch to use, whip for hems and some rips tears, a back stitch, or a long or fine straight stitch.

Moving Things

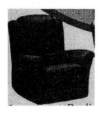

Furniture: My mother always said you had to move furniture in order to vacuum properly. *Okay Mom, we'll do it—single-handedly*!

You *could* simply grab an armchair and drag it out of the way. Inevitably though, dragging will gouge a deep scratch in hard wood or linoleum floors, or tear a hole in the carpet. It's not worth the gamble.

Look at the item you need to move. How can it leverage between your torso/your hip, and the arm you use?

Sometimes, for example lining up your hip with the arm of an armchair, will enable you to pick up the chair by hooking one chair arm over your hip bone and grabbing the other arm with your one hand. I recommend the back of the chair be in front.—it's heavier, and with the back in front, you can keep an eye on it.

Boxes: An oversized but lightweight box can often be managed by squatting down and sliding your open hand, palm up underneath. Wedge the box between your hand and your chin and stand, bringing the box in close to your body.

Setting the table

When you're setting the table just for one or two, you can probably manage carrying the three to eight pieces of flatware in your one hand.

* * * * *

But if you enjoy entertaining, you can try a _utensil basket,_ a basket with a sturdy handle and compartments for the forks, spoons, knives, napkins, etc. I've seen them in dollar stores.

Sweeping

Spot-sweep your linoleum or hardwood floors by crab-walking and swiping at the dust and dirt with a whisk broom.

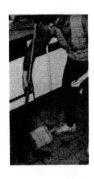

Broom Sweeping: Although two-handed people leverage a broom against the hand holding up high and maneuver it with an _other_ hand down low. Single-handedly, leverage your broom against the shoulder of the hand you use, and maneuver the broom with your one hand. Rest the tip of the broomstick against your collarbone. Wrap the length of your arm along the broomstick so your forearm is on top and your thumb and fingers close naturally around the broom stick. You'll find the broom sweeps better if you leave your index finger stretched long, on top of the broomstick, pointing toward the floor. This helps you reach out with the broom and draw it and the dirt on the floor toward you. Then sweep the dirt into a pile just like anyone else would.

Dustpan

Brace the dustpan, tipping the handle end up with your foot.

You'll find your success at getting everything into the dustpan quickly and more efficiently increases when you squat down and sweep the pile of floor dirt into the dustpan using a whisk brush.

Vacuuming

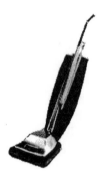

Although vacuuming is primarily a one-handed chore—you only need one hand to pull the equipment and to push the attachment across the floor. Making sure your equipment best suits one-handed use is critical. You don't want a heavy machine either upright or canister. You'll want to make sure that the wheels roll smoothly so the vacuum is easy to push.

* * * * *

The absolute best vacuum equipment is an internal vacuum system. This is a system is built into your home such that the motor and dirt storage are stationary—installed in the garage, a closet, or the basement with tubing installed throughout your house. Wall sockets, into which you plug the vacuum hose, are strategically mounted throughout your home.

An internal vacuum system has no electrical cord to contend with, as it's hard wired into your electrical service The vacuum automatically starts when the hose is fitted into one of the hose sockets, and turns off when the hose is disengaged from the wall socket.

Because you only contend with the hose and attachments, managing this vacuum single-handedly is a breeze.

* * * * *

Alternatively, you want to look for a light weight upright model. Try several in the store showroom. See which works best for you, and do make sure where you buy has a return policy in case that what you thought would work, doesn't. You want to avoid the canister-style vacuum, as pulling the heavy canister, which holds the motor and the dirt storage bag, around behind you can strain your one wrist, elbow, and shoulder.

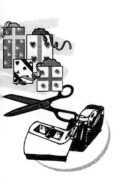

Wrapping gifts

Before you attempt wrapping gifts, you absolutely must have a desk-size cellophane tape dispenser, a large uncluttered table top you can stand at, and, a pair of sharp scissors. Wrapping paper that is folded flat rather than rolled is easier to work with. Likewise, boxed gifts are easier to wrap than oddly shaped packages. So box everything you can, and in preparation, save boxes in the off-season.

An **X-Acto Knife** (*pictured left*) a*vailable in both art and office supply stores*) may cut wrapping paper to size more easily for you single-handedly than do scissors. Cover your table with cardboard to protect it.

Lay the package you want to wrap, in the center of the wrapping paper you want to cut (*with your tape dispenser too if the gift isn't heavy*) to hold the paper while you cut, with the X-Acto Knife or scissors.

Move the tape dispenser within easy reach. If it's a rectangular shape you're wrapping, lift one of the long sides of paper and lay it over top the gift. If it's more of a cube, it doesn't matter where you start. Hold the folded-over paper in place with your forearm and reach for the tape dispenser to set it on the folded-over paper. (*If you can't reach the dispenser, you'd best start again after placing the tape dispenser where you'll be able to reach it while your forearm holds down that first flap of wrapping paper.*)

Once again, hold the folded over paper in place with your forearm, pick up the tape dispenser you moved to an accessible location, and set it down on top of that side of the wrapping paper, so you can

move your arm without the paper un-
wrapping. Now, reach across the package,
lift up the other side of wrapping paper,
bringing it up the other side of the package
and over the top. This piece should also
end a bit more than halfway across the top
side. Slip it under the tape dispenser, then
peel off a piece of tape, and adhere the
tape over the topmost edge in the center of
the package.

After you've taped the two edges together, move the tape dispenser so the cutter edge is close to one of the package
edges that remains unfinished. From the
sides, one at a time, crease the wrapping
paper over the box edge and toward the
center of the side, and crease the paper at
the top and along the bottom.

When you've completed both sides,
you will have two double thickness triangles of wrapping paper sticking out at either box end; one at the top and the other
below. Crease the top flap down so the tip
points at the table. Hold this flap in place
with your thumb. With your ring finger,
reach for the bottom flap catching it—
perhaps with your fingernail. Slide that
bottom flap underneath your thumb.

Shift your hand so your palm is holding
the bottom flap, the tip of which points
toward the ceiling. With your thumb and
index finger now free, reach to the tape
dispenser which you already placed close

to the edge of the box enabling you to pull out and cut off the piece of tape you need.

Just one end left. Repeat what you just accomplished on this end. Move the tape dispenser so the cutter edge is close to the remaining package edge. From the sides, one at a time, crease the wrapping paper over the box edge and toward the center of the side. Now crease the paper at the top and along the bottom. When you've completed both sides, you again have two double thickness triangles of wrapping paper extending from each box end, one at the top and the other at the bottom. Crease the top flap down so that the point is directed at the table. Hold this flap in place with your thumb. With your ring finger, reach for the bottom flap. Slide that bottom flap underneath your thumb. Shift your hand such that your palm is holding the bottom flap, the point of which points toward the ceiling. With your thumb and index finger now free, reach to the tape dispenser to pull out and cut off this last piece of tape.

*   *   *   *   *

You may find that wrapping oddly shaped presents or perhaps any present, is more effort than you want to expend.

Not to worry. Many stores, sell festive gift bags. Before placing your oddly-shaped present into a gift bag, try sitting your gift in the center of a square sheet of tissue paper. Gather the four corners, and twist. Now place your gift inside the gift bag. A small amount of arranging of the tissue paper so it fills the opening of the bag and covers the gift, produces an easily wrapped present that looks stunning!

If you use heavier packaging tape, for which dispensers can also be found, you can use the wrapping procedure above to wrap packages for mailing. Your local U.S. Post Office also sells mailing envelopes and boxes that may more easily fit and better protect what you mail.

Cardboard boxes with flaps.

Cardboard boxes that you've salvaged from where-ever are wonderful for storing off-season stuff—clothing , holiday decorations, etc., for basement and attic storage. But only if you can get them closed.You _could_ tape them shut, but then it's a beast to get inside again. A more suitable solution is to "_weave_" the flaps so the last flap under the corner of the first flap "_locks_" the box shut. This was a trick my Dad's father used. But _he_ had _two_ hands!

Single-handedly, first fold one of the longer flaps down over the open box (_If the flaps are all the same length, because the box is a cube, start with any of the flaps—the one farthest from you will be the easiest._) follow by folding one of the short flaps (_or if the box is a cube, fold one of the flaps adjacent to the first one you folded in_). Next fold in the _other_ long flap (*or for the cube box, flap the adjacent to the last one you folded in*).

Now for the fun part. Fold the last flap over the ends of the long flaps, completely covering the opening of the box (*over the ends of the first and third flaps folded over the opening*). Now lift up the end of the *first* flap, the one you just covered, and slip the end of the short flap underneath, without *unweaving* all the flaps. To do this, rest your elbow on the other end of that last flap as you lift up the corner on the end of that first flap, and slip the end of the last flap underneath.

OFFICEWORK

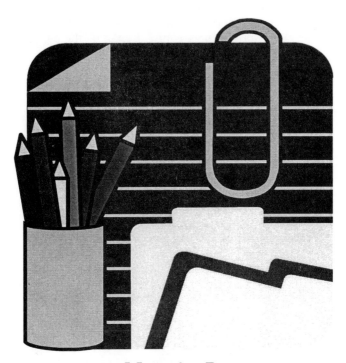

Managing Paper

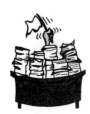

You need to learn about KYDC. **K**eep **Y**our **D**esk **C**lear. We're in the *Information Age*. Even in these days of the *"Paperless Office"* you'll still find yourself managing mountains of paper. And manage it you must, because if you don't you'll be swamped by a paper tidal wave: correspondence, direct mail ads, hard-copy follow-ups of electronic transmissions like e-mail and faxes, newsletters, inter-office memos, basic FYI, and news clips from magazines you've clipped yourself or that come from friends and associates, etc. etc. etc. Conscientiously practicing KYDC is the key to successfully managing the paper morass single-handedly.

Squaring piles of loose paper

You've just gone through an entire file searching for that one piece of information. Now that you've found it, you have to KYDC by stashing the rest of the file back where it came from. You were careful to keep all the pages in order, but now you need to square-off the stack in order to return it to whomever it came from—or get it back into the file drawer.

* * * * *

To square a pile of paper, clear a section of table or desk top. An area of two square feet would be ideal, but just 6" x 14" will do. If the pile of paper at hand is thick, divide it into sections of an inch and a half or so.

About two-thirds down the long edge of the pile, hook your index finger underneath the stack section, with your thumb on top pressed outstretched along the pile of paper. Pull the pages up with your index finger, bending it against your thumb so your middle and ring fingers slip under the stack. Now stand the stack on the other long end, loosely held between your thumb and fingers.

Squeeze your thumb against your fingers, tightening your hold on the stack of paper. Lift the stack off the desk top. Relax your hold on the paper, so the long end taps against the table or desk top, but leave your thumb and fingers in position, bracing the paper. Repeat tapping the section several times.

Press your thumb against your fingers, tightening your hold on the stack of paper and lift the stack off the desk top. and twist your wrist so your thumb points toward the shoulder of the arm you don't use so when you relax our hold, the short end taps against the table top. Repeat the lifting and releasing, tapping the short end on the table top several times.

Lift the stack, rotate your wrist pointing your thumb down to the table top. Relax your hold and tap the long end. Lift the stack, rotate your wrist, your thumb pointing toward the shoulder of the arm you don't use, relax your hold, and tap the short end again. Repeat the rotations two or three or more times, until the stack is squared to your satisfaction.

Signing Letters and Documents

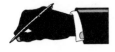

Inevitably, whenever you need to sign a document, your signature goes at the bottom of the page—often so far down the page there isn't enough paper at the bottom to stabilize the page with your one hand palm while your fingers work the ball-point pen through your signature. *Two-handed people use their extra hand to hold the document they're signing.* Single-handedly, you'll need a prop.

When working a your desk, use a **paperweight** kept just for that purpose. The paperweight you choose needs to be heavy enough to stabilize a sheet of paper on a smooth desktop where documents slide around easily. Look for a substantial, but not overly large paperweight.

In a pinch, the stapler will do, but the black rubber bottom may stain white paper—a coffee mug inevitably leaves a coffee stain ring.

* * * * *

If the hand you can't use is your dominant hand, and you can no longer legibly form your signature, using a copy of your signature from before, you can have a **Self-Inking Rubber Signature Stamp** made. By going to your bank or financial institution with this rubber stamp and a copy of something you signed before the accident, you can have your new rubber stamp approved for use on financial documents like your checks. You'll need to be careful not to misplace your signature stamp. Under no circumstances should your bank account number be printed or attached to a signature stamp.

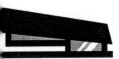

Staples

Staples are an awesome tool for professionals managing single-handedly. Unless you have an *extra* hand to hold a paper clip when you flip through pages, the whole package comes undone. Not so with staples.

You can staple just about every kind of paperwork to help you get it organized. As soon as you open the envelope, staple bills to payment envelopes. Staple itemized register receipts to your credit card receipts. Staple together separate sheets of notes on related subjects. Staple together pieces of correspondence on the same topic, from the same person, or the same company... You get the idea.

Staples are relatively harmless to a document and easily removed as long as you keep a **Staple Remover** handy (*A staple remover is a necessary and inexpensive office accessory for one-handers. Your five fingernails are far too precious to sacrifice on steel staples.*)

You absolutely need a staple remover available *wherever* you do paperwork. If you pay your bills in a different location from where you do other paperwork, indulge yourself with a second or even third stapler and staple remover!

Paper Clips

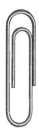

Use paper clips to organize papers *only* if the bundle you're putting together is going to a two-handed someone. One-handedly, paper-clipped papers are hard to manage since they tend to separate, losing the top or the bottom pages. *Funnily enough, two-handed professionals seem to prefer paper clips over staples.*

Binder Clips

Lawyers always use binder clips to clamp together stacks of paper— documents too large to staple. You can too! Binder clips are readily available at most any office supply store, and more economically from the office supply super-stores springing up in and around most the urban areas.

Mail

Mail is a fact of office life sometimes twice a day. There are easy and hard ways to handle it. Hard ways make you feel and look inept. Easy ways won't. So go for easy ways. Sometimes you'll be standing and expected to open an enve-lope right away. Doing so requires a bit of planning. Other times, someone from the mailroom drops mail on your desk; mail you can open more privately.

Envelopes

Opening

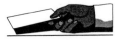

How do you open an envelope without clamping a corner in your teeth? Use the "*First* and *Second Secrets*," B*ody Positioning*, and F*our Fingers and a Thumb*.

While standing:

Press the addressed side of the envelope against your thigh down from your hip bone with the heel of your hand. Trap the envelope perpendicular to the floor. With the heel of your hand pressed against the envelope, about in the middle, slip your index finger under an *ungummed* corner of the flap and start opening the envelope. (*You'll find the edges of the flap are often unglued allowing you to slide your finger inside.*)

With your index finger under the flap, pull your finger toward your palm. Without much effort, you'll lift about four inches of flap away from the envelope.

When your index finger lifting away the flap reaches the heel of your hand, press the tip of your ring finger into the envelope, trapping the envelope against your body while keeping your index finger under the flap. Lift and slide your palm, back, so you *inch-worm* your palm along the sealed edge of the envelope. Straighten your index finger and go back to lifting the flap away from the envelope.

Draw your index finger toward your palm again and continue lifting the flap away from the envelope. Keep pulling down and *inch-worming* toward the palm of your hand until you've fully pulled away the flap.

Now you only need to get at the contents of the envelope. Press your index finger into the center of the envelope (*both center left to right and center top to bottom*) Only your index finger is pressing the envelope against your thigh. Then slide the palm of your hand down toward the floor, in line with your index finger.

Slide the palm of your hand back up, opening the flap and stretch out your thumb. Stop sliding when your palm is over the gummed edge of the flap. Now, the palm of your hand and your wrist trap the envelope against your body.

Slip your index finger into the envelope, opening the envelope wide allowing you to get inside by pressing your thumb into the flap and stretching your index finger out.

With palm and wrist still trapping the envelope, slip your middle finger inside the envelope beside your index finger and begin removing the contents of the envelope between your index finger and thumb. Raise your wrist, pulling the contents halfway out of the envelope.

By rolling your forearm toward the floor so your hand turns over on your pinkie finger, pressing the heel of your hand against the envelope again, and sliding your middle, index, and pinkie fingernails along the envelope, stretch down your fingers pinching the envelope between your ring and middle fingers.

Ta-da

A flick of the wrist shakes the letter open for reading. *You can become so adept at this procedure that you won't even need to watch your hand perform, you'll just keep on talking to whomever it was that handed the envelope to you, or anyone else who might walk by, just like two-handed people. Folks will hardly be aware of what you're doing.*

While sitting

If you're seated, you can open an envelope either by trapping it against your thigh and following the same procedure you used standing. Or, lay it flat on the desk, flap side up. Rest your index finger so it slides underneath the flap, and trap the envelope with your thumb halfway down the flap, near the edge, and pinkie finger in the middle of the bottom edge.

This method can be done on a flat table, but is easier with a beveled edge, enabling you to brace the envelope while working. Without the beveled edge, sit closer and use your abdomen for leverage.

If you slide your index finger down the length of the gummed flap, all the while holding the envelope steady with your thumb and index finger, very shortly, you'll have opened the envelope. Press your index finger into the middle of the envelope, under the flap and pivot your hand over the envelope your middle finger opening the flap. Press your middle finger down on the flap, trapping the envelope. Now you can slide your index finger and thumb inside the envelope to pull out the contents. ***Done!***

Alternatively, while seated, you can use a letter opener if you trap the envelope, flap side up, between your knees. With your one hand manning the letter opener, slash the flap. Put down the opener, and pull out the contents of the envelope. Sitting is so much easier...

Stuffing

Fold the letter pages in thirds. Firmly crease the folds with your thumbnail by trapping the page at the fold with your middle finger, and scraping your thumb nail down the fold.

Fold the envelope flap back so it lies flat. Sit close enough to the edge of your desk to leverage the bottom of the envelope against your abdomen or chest and slide the contents inside.

Organization

Setting up systems to organize the information you need to perform your job effectively, so it's close at hand is critical. Sticking to your systems keeps you on track for success in a business environment *expecting* everyone to be, *or to function as if they are*, two-handed.

Filing

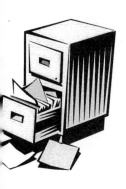

Is it *anyone's* favorite subject? Nonetheless in order to manage paper single-handedly, spending some time to develop, to establish, and then maintain an effective system is essential. Single-handedly you can't afford to let paper get ahead of you. What you aren't working on at the moment needs to be stashed where you can find it when you need it.

* * * * *

Hanging file folders are invaluable in that by using manila folders inside, you can remove the manila folder with the papers you need, leaving the hanging file folder in the drawer, marking the manila file's location. Manila folders make it easy to segregate paperwork on your desk while working on multiple projects simultaneously, and to return documents to the right drawer after finishing with them.

Telephone books

No office is complete without a full set of local and metropolitan-area white and yellow pages phone books, zip code directories, and appropriate industry catalogs. These books tend to be large, soft-covered, thin paged and cumbersome. With one hand you need to plan how to organize and store directories.

If you try standing your directories and catalogs upright on a shelf, you need to pack them in quite tightly else they don't stay upright. And if they're packed too closely, they're nearly impossible to return after using them.

Not only do the pages of the directory you want to return splay open when you pick it up so it won't slide easily into place, but the rest of the directories seem to *exhale*, taking up more space. You can try opening space for the directory you've used by pulling adjacent directories forward a bit and wedging your directory back into place. Inevitably though, one cover folds over and then tears...

* * * * *

If you stack your directories horizontally, reaching for the bottom directory can mean an avalanche, or worse yet a strain injury in your one hand as you try to prevent that avalanche.

* * * * *

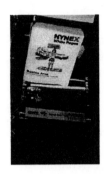

Instead, try storing directories and catalogs in a hanging file drawer beside you. Rack them in the drawer like hanging files by scavenging the metal bars from old hanging file folders and slipping a bar into the center of each directory. These bars are designed to straddle a file drawer, so when you open the drawer, You'll be looking down on the labeled spines of all your directories. This way, you can quickly select the one you need. It's almost easy to follow Rule #1 KYDC. Since the directories smoothly slide back into place, you'll put them away.

Pencils

I use pencils all the time to: *Mark my calendar*—how often do ironclad dates get rescheduled? *Label computer disks*—erasing the old label after reformatting recycles, *Mark file folder labels*—erasing the old label recycles folders after old paper files are discarded in the recycling bin.

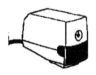

Unlike pens, for which the ink seems to flow almost endlessly, pencils loose their point after a few words. Fortunately, unlike a pen out of ink, you can sharpen a dull pencil.

To single-handedly sharpen pencils, you need an electric sharpener. Most offices have one, but if yours doesn't, it's an inexpensive reasonable accommodation under ADA (*Americans with Disabilities Act of 1990, Public Law 101-336*).

Computers

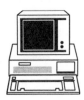

Organization is the perfect segue to computers. If you embrace technology, it will enable you to function in a business or leisure environment as effectively as two-handed people. Just learn to hand over as much as possible to the machine.

By embracing technology, computers become your *tools*, freeing you to do the creative thinking, only you can do, leaving the machine to implement your thoughts

Probably your most difficult step will be convincing an employer that you can single-handedly manage the job you want. The best way to do that is to regain confidence in your abilities through experience. Get that experience by owning your own equipment, through classes, by using friends' equipment or machines available to the public at many libraries and community colleges. You'll want to become comfortable with computers by getting to know the basics of the hardware, but only the hardware you'll use.

Just as you don't need to know about carburetors and spark plugs to drive a car (only the ignition, knobs and dials on the dash, steering wheel, and the pedals) you don't need to know much about your computer's innards. You need only know how to turn it on, how to get data into it (*via keyboard, scanner, modem, floppy and CD-drives*) and how to get data out of it (*via printer, modem, floppy disks, tape drive*) and about various software packages that enable you to accomplish your tasks. *It sounds like a lot, but it really isn't.*

Hardware

Hardware refers to the metal, plastic, and glass components you use to compute. Basic hardware includes the monitor, keyboard, and tower or desktop *box* housing the CPU (*Central Processing Unit*), the hard drive, floppy disk disks, and CD-ROM drive. Hardware also includes *peripherals* like speakers, printers, modems, scanners, and so on.

Keyboards

QWERTY

If you once typed with two hands you already know the QWERTY keyboard. That's part of the process. If you never typed before, your first responsibility is to learn your way around a keyboard. You'll learn by practicing, w*hich is, as my German teacher once told us (in German), the way you get to Carnegie Hall...*

Start the learning before you have access to a computer by bringing your typing up to speed on a typewriter. Computer keyboards have a few more keys, but the central, alpha-numeric and symbol input keys are the same. Once you've got those typewriter keys down, adding the extra computer-specific keys won't be difficult.

Why not start by typing correspondence on a typewriter. The faster you are on the keyboard, the more effective your computing skills will be.

If your work involves ideas coming directly from your head, as opposed to copy-typing, it's okay to look at the keyboard watching your fingers most of the time. Knowing your way around the keyboard so you're not wasting time searching for keys will speed your progress.

If you need to *transcribe your or someone else's words*, it *can* be done, although it's slower since the only way to do it is to read and memorize a half dozen words, look down at the keyboard, enter each letter, one-by-one, look back at the copy and read the next half dozen words... The more you do, the faster you become.

New!

If teaching yourself one-handed typing isn't working, Take a look at Nina Richardson's *Type with One Hand*, ISBN 05386 82752. This thirty-two page book shows you a functional approach, helping you improve both speed and accuracy. (*See* **Resources**, *page 246.*

New!

Another option is *Half-QWERTY*, a software program that enables you to type fluidly using only one half of the normal full-size keyboard. The *Matias Corporation*, developer of this system, reports typing speeds of 64 words-per-minute. (*See Resources Index, Page 246*)

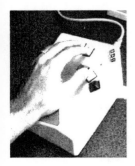

If the hand you use isn't your dominant hand, you may find a full keyboard daunting. *Infogrip*, Inc's **Personal Keyboard**. was specifically designed for one-handed use. The keyboard consists of seven comfortably laid out keys. When using the **Personal Keyboard**, your palm rests on an ergonomically correct palm support. Your thumb roves between three keys, while each finger is responsible for a single key. Letters, numbers, and symbols are entered by pressing a pre-determined or self-programmed combination of keys with the fingers of your one hand (*See* **Resources**, *Page 246*.)

Foot Pedals

Another way to help manage keying in data single-handedly, is to add **Step On It** computer control foot pedals to the hardware on your machine. Plugged into your computer equipment between the CPU (*Central Processing Unit*) and your keyboard, a foot pedal can be configured to replace the Ctrl, Alt or Shift keys, or any other frequently used keystroke combinations of your choice, like combinations that are *outside the span* of your one hand see **Resources**, *Page 246*.)

Scanners

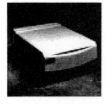

Scanning technology has improved so it is now possible to feed hardcopy text into a desktop scanner for your computer to *transcribe"* into a digital file, enabling you to incorporate the scanned file into other documents, or for storage. Scanning can help you manage paper documents you used to file, or can even take-over your transcription tasks.

Companies market scanning equipment, ranging from hand-held models, enabling you to manually select text or images you want scanned, to flatbed scanners (*pictured above*), used similar to photocopiers except instead of generating paper, scanners generate digital files from a paper document to save on your computer hard disk.

Software

Software is the part of computing that instructs your computer hardware in performing the tasks you bought it to do. The software is the computer's capability.

The more software applications you're familiar with, the more uses you'll have for your personal computer. What follow are a number of software categories and names of top-selling (*but not necessarily the best*) titles in each category. Depending on what you want to do with your computer, you'll want to sample at least one software title from several categories.

Accounting

Things have come a long way since the days of green eye-shades, ledger books and pencils. As small, medium, and as start-up companies take accounting in-house with accounting software, learning an accounting software package becomes all the more important to your career. Top-selling software include: *Peachtree Accounting*, Intuit *Quickbooks*, BestWare *MYOB*, and *CheckMark* Software *MultiLedger*.

Contact Management

Also known as *Personal Information Managers (PIMs)*, **Contact Management Software** enables you to computerize your *"to-do"* list, your appointment schedule, your address book, as well as to integrate phone call lists task lists, and master plan list for those long-term projects you're chunking away at on a day-by-day basis. *Contact Management Software* enables you to gather together and consolidate notes and data you've learned about people with whom you've spoken or intend to contact—improving efficiency by reducing your need to rely on memory.

Instead of shoveling through dozens of handwritten notes *Contact Management Software* helps you put it all together. Top-selling packages in this category include: *Sidekick* from Starfish, *TouchBase*, *Goldmine*, and Symantecs' *Act!*.

Database

Database software allows you to create *three-dimensional spreadsheets (see page 195).* Because of it's flexibility, Database software has become wildly popular in business. Top-selling database packages include: Lotus *Approach*, *FileMaker Pro* for Macintosh, and Microsoft *Access*.

DeskTop Publishing/Page Layout

Like *Database* and *Presentation* Software **DeskTop Publishing Software** which enables the design of high-quality collateral's (*brochures, hand-outs, newsletters, and late-breaking news sheets, etc.*) has become popular in business. Some of the top-selling **DeskTop Publishing** packages include: Adobe *Page-Maker*, *QuarkXPress*, and as an entry-level, alternative, Microsoft *Publisher*.

Financial Management

Whether you're a *"technical"* investor (*comparing historical market trends and movements*) or a *"value"* investor (*collecting tidbits of news on specific companies that interest you*), your PC can replace pencil, eraser, graph paper, notebooks, calculator, and a library of books. By inputting your portfolio data, or investment opportunities you want to track, you can stay on top as efficiently as a financial services professional. Top selling financial management programs include: *Quicken* from Intuit, *Managing Your Money*, and Microsoft *Money*.

Optical Character Recognition (OCR)

OCR software works with a scanner to translate scanned text into editable digital files (*text files you can manipulate with your Word-Processing Software (see page 197)*). Top-selling OCR software include: Xerox *TextBridge*, CyberVision *Type Reader*, *Adobe Capture*, and Caere *OmniPage*.

Presentation

Presentation software enables you to design integrated audio visual aids to accompany informational, training, and sales presentations. Companies now look for employees capable of preparing their own presentation aids using presentation software. Top-selling packages include: *Lotus Freelance Graphics, Harvard Graphics*, and *Microsoft PowerPoint*

Spreadsheets

In developing business skills, you should get used to using **Spreadsheets**. Once you have, you'll wonder how you ever managed without computer spreadsheets. Organizing data in spreadsheets can be incredibly time-saving, even addicting. Just as with word processing there are many inexpensive less-widely used packages. But because of their popularity in business, you probably want to familiarize yourself with one of the top-selling ones such as: Lotus 1-2-3, *Microsoft Excel,* and *Borland Quattro Pro.*

Utilities

Several Software Utility packages from a number of different companies enable you to execute commands requiring the simultaneous depression of multiple keys. Keys that need to be pressed together aren't always adjacent, and often lie outside the span of your one hand. You can manage by adding the so-called "*Sticky Key*" utility to your machine. Makers and titles of this *must-have* utility include: *Microsoft "Access"* (*not to be confused with Microsoft's database program of the same name*), *Sticky-Key* from *MicroSystems* and *ProKey* from *RoseSoft*.

Voice Recognition

As American business fixates on "*downsizing,*" often by paring down support staffs, executives are finding they need to handle more of their own clerical work. Many of these executives never learned to type. Thus *Voice Recognition* computer equipment—once an adaptation for people with disability—has gained greater notice and increased funding.

That's good news for those of us managing single-handedly. You *can* learn to type with one hand fast enough for most of your needs, but as you do more with your computer, you may find typing speed is the limiting factor. Luckily, Voice Recognition software is approaching both affordability and accuracy.

It used to be that voice recognition software required you to speak oh so slowly—like HAL in "*2001: A Space Odys-*

sey." Already several programs allow "continuous number" input, making numerical data-entry doable. It won't be long before you'll be able to talk words into your computer as easily as you talk into a tape recorder. The only difference being, with Voice Recognition, the computer will translate your words into editable text you can manipulate and print.

Word-Processing

This is the software that enables your computer to manipulate text. Most people, at least part of the time, use a personal computer for writing. Although there are many word-processing software packages on the market, if you're seeking marketable business skills, it's probably wise to learn one of the top selling packages rather than a cheaper and perhaps more limited word-processing software. These top-selling word-processing packages include: Microsoft *Word*, Borland *WordPerfect*, Lotus *Ami-Pro*.

Newspaper Clipping

At first glance, scissors might seem to be something you can easily manage single-handedly. That is, until you find out how much holding your *other* hand is supposed to be doing.

This is not an insurmountable problem. You simply need to have the right props handy. In this instance, the right props include a clear flat surface (*an uncluttered desk or table*) and a *Heavy Something* such as a paperweight, ceramic mug, your tape dispenser or stapler.

Spread the document to be clipped, flat on the table. You'll often find it easier to stand when cutting single-handedly. Standing improves your perspective, making for a neater job.

Set your *"Heavy Something"* on the page to be clipped, not within the article, but a few inches outside the perimeter. As you cut, move your *"Heavy Something,"* adjusting placement as you proceed.

Another option for *"clipping"* smaller items, things like the *help wanteds* and other classifieds, is to firmly outline the ad in ink using a ball-point pen. The scoring of the pen breaks the paper as if you'd perforated it, enabling you to remove the ad as if cut with a scissors.

* * * * *

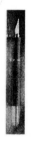

Alternatively, try an *X-Acto Knife,* (*pictured left*) typically used to lay-out advertising art, or architectural drawings. It's a razor blade attached to a pen-like handle. Use an X-Acto knife to score around whatever it is you wish to cut out.

Phones

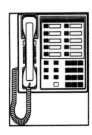

You *can* manage a telephone single-handedly. If you think about it, it only takes one hand to pick up the receiver. Once you've done that, it's only natural to clench the receiver between your shoulder and your ear, freeing up your *one* hand for dialing or writing, picking up your coffee, whatever—for a while anyway.

Headsets

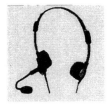

A telephone headset allows you to wear the telephone receiver on your head like ear muffs It not only frees your one hand for other tasks, but also helps you to maintain proper posture while you work with the phone. If you use the phone a lot, you can choose to wear the headset *all the time,* disconnecting it from the phone when you need to leave your work area, or you could take off the headset, putting it back on when you return.

Speaker phones

A speaker phone is another way to free your one hand while working on the telephone. A few drawbacks: voice quality of speaker phones isn't as clear, and your conversation privacy is greatly diminished. You often get a speaker phone "*base*" with a cordless phone. That way, when the receiver is elsewhere, one can answer the base/speaker phone.

Phone Dialers

If juggling the telephone receiver, a computer keyboard, and telephone touch-pad simultaneously, or even one after the other single-handedly, proves too much you can have your phone dialed for you by your computer, or by an electronic phone dialer. Your phone dialer can be pocket-sized, or a larger desktop model.

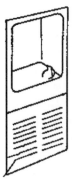

Water Coolers

Usually it's sufficient just to press the button with your one hand, lean over, and slurp from the fountain. But what if you want to fill a cup and bring some of that filtered water back to your desk?

Hold the cup in your one hand, either by wrapping your fingers around it, or if it's a mug, by the handle. With your fore-arm over the water fountain button, bend your wrist to about a 90° angle so the cup is approximately under the line of the water flow. Press your forearm onto the button. Adjust the positioning of your cup, and Voile! Water in a cup!

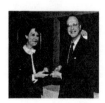

Accepting an Award

You've been chosen to receive an award. *Congratulations!* So, you're preparing for a formal event complete with stage, audience, photographer, and an *important someone* presenting.

When two-handed people accept awards they use both hands—one to reach for the award the other to simultaneously shake hands with the *important someone.*

As soon as possible, single-handed-you needs to approach both the presenter and the photographer. Your case is a bit different, and these people need to be prepared. Tell them you use one hand.

Explain that to receive your award, you will first smile and shake the presenter's hand. Then, still smiling, you will release the handshake and reach with the *same* hand for the award. Suggest pausing and posing for pictures both at the handshake and at receiving the award. Preferably the presenter will choose to present the award to you with both hands and not rest his/her *other hand* on your shoulder.

If you're supposed to make some remarks, turn toward the microphone and speak. Otherwise simply walk off the stage, smiling all the way across.

Who knows, maybe you'll be awarded after reading this book, for successfully managing single-handedly!

TRAVELING

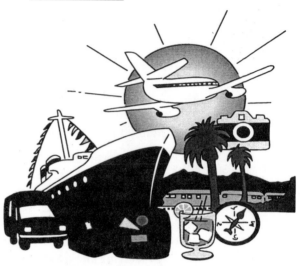

Of course you can travel single-handedly. It just involves a bit more planning.

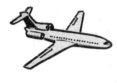

Air Travel

When traveling by air, make sure your travel agent completes *advance check-in* and *seat selections* when making your reservations.

Seat Selection If you travel economy class, you do *not* want a seat in the first row behind the First Class section. While these seats offer more leg room, they don't have the tray table dropping from the back of the seat in front of you—*there is no seat in front of you*—only the wall separating

Economy from First Class. The tray tables for these seats pull up from the arm of your seat, an arrangement isn't easily managed single-handedly.

Aisle seats are preferable to window or center seats, they're roomier and easier to access. You'll want to choose the aisle seat with the arm you use on the aisle. This way you protect your *other* arm/hand from passengers and flight crew passing by. Also, with the hand you use on the outside, it's easier to get up, to use the facilities or for leg stretching.

So if you use your right hand, choose an aisle seat on the right side of the row of seats. If you use your left hand, choose an aisle seat on the left.

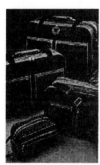

Luggage When traveling single-handedly, bring minimal luggage. Now is the time to learn *the fine art of packing light,* especially since you'll need to bring a select few of your gadgets. Purchase carry-on **luggage with wheels and a handle**, that fits under your seat. You *don't* want to use overhead compartments. People cram the most amazing things into those compartments—things which shift around during flight. You do not want to be rummaging overhead with your one hand, unable to protect yourself from the bowling ball in a canvass bag careening toward you.

Early Boarding When the flight crew announces early boarding for families with children, seniors, and people with disability, *step in line*. This early boarding enables you to take the more time necessary to arrange your things and settle yourself in comfortably, without inconveniencing passengers behind you.

Airplane restrooms are tiny and hard to maneuver in. Even so, grab bars are liberally located throughout. *Use the grab bars*. You've probably already noticed how much losing the use of a hand or arm has affected your balance. When using an airplane restroom, you'll be trying to steady yourself in a cramped space that's moving and frequently bumping. Think of it this way, *no one will ever know if you stayed on your feet because of a grab bar, but they'll all know you don't*.

Inevitably, you'll find you'll need to plan ahead because the toilet paper dispenser's mounted on the *wrong side* for your one hand. Prepare for this in advance. Tear off the paper you'll need, and stash it in a pocket, *before* you sit down.

Typically, sink water in airplane restrooms only flows from the faucets when the handle is depressed. To get around this problem, rinse out the sink, push down the stopper, then fill the sink with enough water to wash your hand.

If your plane encounters turbulence while you're in the restroom, stay seated, finish up as best you can, and pull together your clothes as quickly as possible, Steadying yourself with a grab bar. If you feel you're in trouble, press the *flight attendant call button*. Flight crew are trained to assist passengers out of the restrooms during turbulence.

Car Travel

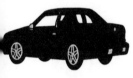

Losing the use of a hand or arm does not mean losing the ability to drive. Many learn to drive safely and legally with one hand.

If your disabilities are more complicated than *"just"* a hand or arm, you need to assess whether cognitive or sensory abilities, needed to drive safely, have also affected.

For obvious reasons, you' can quickly see that *Standard Shift Transmissions* while *doable*, are difficult single-handedly. Do the benefits of the manual shift outweigh the added difficulties of operating it?

Several companies, for-profit and non-profit, specialize in enabling people with disability to drive using adaptations for cars. Each of the major American car companies has made substantial commitment to adaptive driving equipment.

* * * * *

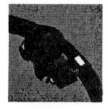

A ***Steering Wheel Knob*** is commonly added a vehicle to help people drive with one hand. Attached to the steering wheel, the knob helps you complete turns. Additional mirrors may also be helpful, for example, if you find it difficult to turn your head to watch through the rear window when backing.

Train and Bus Travel

Once again, whenever you travel, make your reservations and pay for them in advance. When traveling, you're trying to keep track of more stuff than usual. The less often you reach for your wallet to handle money single-handedly while hanging onto your stuff, the better.

As always, you want to pack as little as possible, no matter how far you're going. All trips up to a week duration, are candidates for packing a single piece of wheeled "*carry-on*" luggage with a handle that can be easily pulled along behind you. For longer trips, try to find wheeled luggage that you can maneuver effectively single-handedly. Try pulling the various pieces of luggage around in the store. But remember, the empty luggage in the store doesn't weigh what it will packed, especially after you've been schlepping it around for a few days.

It's easiest if the seat beside you is empty and you can lay your one bag on that empty seat, enabling you to take out the book or whatever project you brought to amuse yourself during the trip. Alternatively, some bus seats are designed similar to airplane seats with space to stow luggage under the seat in front of you. If not, have the driver stash your bag in the luggage compartment underneath.

You don't want to use the overhead luggage racks. Single-handedly reaching up overhead for your bag—even a small carry-on—leaves you vulnerable to an avalanche of other people's luggage when you try pulling yours free during or at the end of the trip.

Even though the restrooms in buses and trains tend to be small, you may find the toilet paper on the *wrong side*. Prepare ahead by tearing off the paper you'll need and stashing it in an accessible pocket *before* you sit down.

Typically, water in bus and train restrooms flows from the faucet only when the handle is depressed. Get around this by rinsing out the sink, pushing down the stopper, and filling the sink with enough water to wash your one hand.

HOUSEHOLD REPAIRS

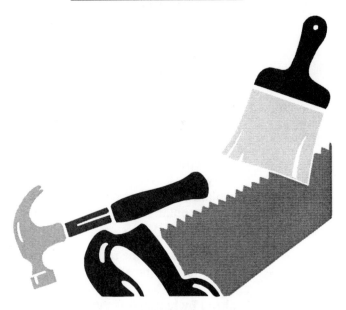

You can still manage many household projects and repairs, single handedly. My grandfather, Duke, (*see page 5*) did a lot of the finish work on his boat, and fixed many things around the house. And me, I've stripped, stained, and polyurethaned all the woodwork in my home as well as quite a bit of furniture. I've also hung pictures, hammered countless nails, sawed, drilled, screwed-in screws, performed *open toilet,* and even some open computer *surgery,* all single-handedly.

You can too!

The right Stuff

Linemen, working on electrical tower lines and atop ladders, way above ground-level bring every tool they could possibly need strapped to their body on a tool belt, or stashed in the pockets of their clothes. Linemen's work clothing is typically designed with many deep pockets. If you're going to successfully manage household maintenance single-handedly, you need to consider these things. Choose work clothing with generous pockets, and consider wearing a tool belt.

Handling Equipment

By keeping the *Three Secrets* in mind (*body positioning, four fingers and a thumb*, and *gadgets*) you can figure out how to accomplish most projects. I've finished woodwork for six, six-foot windows, seven door frames, four dressers, a four foot by 15" by 15" three-door cabinet among other wood finishing projects, with stain and polyurethane. But when it came to hanging that cabinet, I decided to seek out another pair of hands, and was the *"third"* one. That's okay. I did a nice job finishing the cabinet, a beautiful job finishing the mop board in every room of my home, dressers, shelves and a bunch of other stuff—all of it single-handedly.

Nails

When hammering into a horizontal plane, start by taking the nail between your thumb, index and middle fingers. Press the point of the nail into whatever it's to nail into *(wall, length of wood, whatever)*.

If you press and twist the nail, you'll begin a nail hole, allowing you to release the nail shaft while the nail stays in place, balanced by its tip in the nail hole beginning you made manually. Now tap the nail lightly and squarely on the head, beginning to drive the nail into its destination. By tapping carefully and squarely, the nail will remain upright. Tap again, and again, each time a bit more firmly as more of the nail tip embeds. After a few taps, the nail tip will go in enough allowing you to firmly strike, driving in the nail.

* * * * *

You can also try using your power drill (see *page 212*), and a drill bit smaller than the nail you're working with. Just *start* the hole, such that the drill bit barely bites into the wood. Then stick the nail tip in the *hole-start*. Press against the nail, getting it to stand, then hammer progressively as above. Tap with your hammer squarely on the head, but lightly at first.

* * * * *

If you're driving a nail into a vertical plane, the tip needs to press more deeply into the wood than for a horizontal, but it _can_ be done.

Picture Hooks

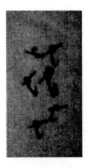

If you can drive a nail, see **Nails** above, you can manage the tack nail and picture hook you got at the hardware store, and get your new _wall art off the floor and_ hung.

First, holding the tack nail near the head, "_press twist_" the point into the wall where the picture is to be hung, beginning a hole. When the hole is deep enough that when you let go of the tack nail it remains sticking into the wall, carefully pull the tack nail out of the hole, trying not to disturb the paint and sheet rock around the hole. Slip the tack nail through the holes in the picture hook with the tack nail point protruding out the back, as it will when the hook is affixed to the wall.

Stick the tack nail with hook back attached into hole beginning, again being careful not to chip surrounding paint or sheet rock. With the end of the tack nail stuck into the hole, let the hook slide down the shaft of the tack nail. Still holding the hook pressed against the wall, press your index finger against the head of the tack nail to more firmly seat the tack nail point in the wall. Slowly release your hold on the hook.

If it feels as though it won't hold, press your index finger against the tack nail head again. Once the nail holds, lightly tap the tack nail head with your hammer. Tap the tack nail head flush against the picture hook, the nail shaft fully embedded in the wall.

Power drill

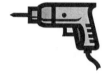

You can operate a power drill single-handedly. Just make sure that the model you've chosen to use is well balanced and not too heavy. All you need to do is grip the drill by its handle, line up the tip of the drill bit square to the surface you're drilling into. Depress the power switch and lean into the handle firmly enough to ease the drill bit into the surface.

The adaptations come with changing (*withdrawing, and inserting*) the drill bit. All you need to do here is remember the First Secret, *Body Positioning see page 11.* Clamp the drill firmly between your knees so the drill chuck points up at you. You may find it easier to sit down in order to comfortably pick up the chuck key in your one hand. Set the tip of the chuck key into its keyhole lining up the chuck key teeth in the chuck gears. Twist the chuck key to loosen the jaws *just* enough to slide in the chosen drill bit.

If you open the jaws too widely, when you tighten down the jaws, the drill bit will list from side to side, and be more difficult to fix in the jaws squarely.

Push the drill bit between the jaws. If it slides in too easily, flopping side to side, remove the drill bit, take up the chuck key again, and close down the jaws enough just to push the drill bit in.

With the drill bit stuck amongst the jaws, pick up your chuck key again and firmly tighten down the jaws, clamping the bit. Now you're ready to make those holes and get going on that project!

Saw

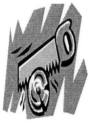

Of course it only takes one hand to grip a saw by its handle to push and pull back and forth through the wood you're cutting. The adaptations come with how you *hold* steady what you cut while you saw.

For small jobs you can install a vise in your work area. For larger projects, a two-by-four for example, you'll want to call on the First Secret, *Body Positioning* (*see page 11*). You need something to lay the two-by-four on. Milk crates, easily relocated and sturdily constructed, work well for this. Lay the two-by-four across your milk crate, using two if you need for the length. Step on the two-by-four to hold it in place, fairly close to where you want to make the cut, but far enough away to allow you to comfortably draw the saw through the wood. Now saw. With the 2x4 anchored by your body weight through your foot, you can get started on those home improvement projects!

Scraper

It's really nothing more than a metal handle for a old-fashioned double edged razor blade, but a Scraper is a *must-have* tool for the single-handed toolbox. It enables you to accomplish a myriad of projects: When paint strays off your brush onto the window pane, drying before you can put down the brush and wipe with your turpentine soaked rag, When polyurethane drips on the "other side—escaping notice until dried solid, When you discover glue has dribbled off the glue bottle nozzle drying onto a finished surface before you could wipe...

Not to worry!

A scraper is designed to resolve these *indiscretions,* making your single-handed projects look as good as anyone else's. After watching you work, your two-handed friends be will be adding a scraper to their own toolboxes.

Painting

 Small painting projects probably won't seem all that different single-handedly, from what they were with two-hands. As long as you organize your materials within easy reach, one-handed painting won't be a problem, but for not having an *other* hand to spell your one had with. With your one hand, arm, and shoulder doing all the work you'll need more frequent breaks.

Because your sense of balance is impacted by one-handedness, you'll find large painting projects—using a paint tray and roller on walls and ceilings, for example, more difficult to get used to. If your one-handedness is temporary, do yourself a favor—postpone the project until you heal.

If your one-handedness is long-term, you need to first work with your physical therapist to re-establish your equilibrium in light of your new circumstances. Once you've taken care of the balance issues, you're ready to get down to work.

Choose painting clothes with generous pockets for stashing things while you paint, arrange your materials within easy reach, and establish _"staging locations"_ where you can put things down—the paint can, your paintbrush, a rag or two, etc. Once you get your center of balance and your equipment organized, go nuts...

Living room need a coat of paint? You can take care of it, single-handedly!

OUTSIDE HOME

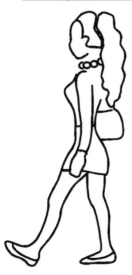

Carrying Things

Two-handed people can afford to waste a hand carrying disorganized armfuls of stuff. If an item starts to slip or fall, they have that *other* hand to catch it and straighten things out. Because we haven't that flexibility. Single-handedly, we must plan ahead in order to successfully manage our loads of miscellaneous (*paper, groceries, purchases, and* just basic *stuff*).

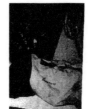

Sacks & Bags

First, add to your supply of canvass bags. Bags with straps long enough to carry the bag over the shoulder of the arm you use to relieve your wrist and forearm while you carry your load. These longer straps should loop at least 10", from the top of the bag. With these, you can slip one strap off your shoulder to open the bag, allowing you to reach inside with your one hand to grab the reading you brought for the subway, or that document for a colleague.

Whenever you go out—shopping for groceries or clothing, or just out, always bring a canvass bag. If you also bring a knapsack stuffed into your canvass bag, you can single-handedly manage the equivalent of two grocery bags.

Keep a plastic shopping bag in the coat pocket you don't use (*the one on the side of the hand you don't use.*) That way, you can manage the stuff inevitably collected whenever you're out. Or stash a plastic shopping bag in your briefcase.

Pocketbooks & purses

Hand Bags When there's so much else you need your one hand to do, why fill it up carrying a handbag? Even with the handle over your wrist, handbags are still in the way.

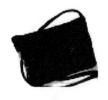

Shoulder bags, slung over your head so the strap crosses your chest and the pocketbook rests on the same hip as the hand you use, leave your one hand free for the obstacles of getting around—doors to open, walk light signal buttons to press, friend ands acquaintances to greet, etc. With your one hand so active, you'll be freer if you don't just drape the strap over the shoulder of the arm you use. With your shoulder bag strap diagonally across your chest, it's also easy to dig for your keys, wallet, tissue, lipstick, etc.

Briefcases You'll be more effective if you carry your briefcase using the shoulder strap crossed from the shoulder of the hand you don't use, to the hip on the side of the hand you do use.

Fanny Packs are the ultimate pocketbook solution for one-handeders. With your essentials strapped around your waist, when you need to get inside just swing the pouch in front, zip it open, and dig inside. The bag attached to your waist gives you leverage to work against, allowing you to retrieve what you need, and to zip the bag closed again.

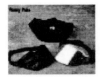

It used to be *fanny packs* were only available in few colors of boat canvass. Not any more! Now you can find beaded fanny packs for evening wear, leather fanny packs for office wear, and every-day packs in nylon, vinyl, and canvass.

Covering Your Ears

Standing below ground on the subway platform, waiting for the next train, I was overwhelmed by the deafeningly loud high-pitched squeal of a train rounding a bend on the other track. There was no where to hide to escape the noise. All around me two-handed subway riders covered their ears with their two hands.

I allowed my self to wallow in self-pity for a moment—until I thought: *Of course! The first secret, body positioning.*

oto by JoAnne N. Mayer

You can cover your ears and protect yourself from deafening noises: **1)** shrug the shoulder of the arm you use up and tip your head into it. **2)** Wrap the arm you use over your head, pressing the round of your shoulder into that ear. **3)** Press the palm of your one hand over the ear on the side of your *other* hand.

This method works as effectively as covering the ears with two hands. I've even watched as two-handed people *with one hand full* gratefully copied my method to block loud noise they couldn't escape.

Mailboxes

Mailboxes are designed to be used with two hands. Two-handed people hold their mail in one hand and pull the swinging door open with their *other* hand.

Not to worry! Mailboxes *can* be managed single handedly. Just remember the **Third Secret—*four fingers and a thumb.*"** Hold eight or ten envelopes pinched between your thumb and index finger at the stamped corner, leaving your middle, ring, and pinkie fingers free. Hook your pinkie over the mailbox door handle, and pull the door open as wide as it'll go. Flip your wrist over so the envelopes rest on the opened mailbox door, more onto the door than off. Unhook your pinkie finger—letting the door begin to close, so the envelopes slide in and down into the box.

* * * * *

Also, use this same method to return library books and videos after-hours, and for making those late-night bank deposits.

Elastic Bands

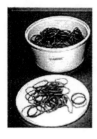

With two hands, elastic bands are handy for many purposes—*organizing and storing seasonal stuff, straightening up the kitchen, arranging the study, out in the workshop, almost anywhere.* Single-handedly, without an *other hand* to bundle together what you're banding while you stretch the elastic band, it might seem impossible.

It isn't.

You can manage elastic bands both while seated, or when standing. One or the other position may be more comfortable for you, so try it both ways.

With the hand you use, gather together the items you want to band. Try this first with easily managed stuff like half dozen butter knives. Squeeze the bundle together between your knees with enough of one end sticking out for your one hand to wrap the elastic band around. You can also try sitting on the floor and clamping the items to be banded between your feet, like a chimpanzee. With the items bunched together, wrap the band around the *"sticking out"* end.

Checkbooks

You may have found yourself with the check you've just written not tearing out along the perforated line—*when the perforations just don't seem to work for you single-handedly.* Resolve this problem, by lifting the check and folding it back along the perforations. You can also run your index finger along the perforations to further weaken the paper. Flatten the check back in place.

Now, holding the bottom right corner of the check you just wrote, between your thumb and middle finger. Stretch your index finger up and press it down on the check book binding.

Rest your pinkie and ring fingers on the blank checks underneath and pull down with your middle finger and thumb. Your index finger on the binding and ring and pinkie fingers on the check underneath should anchor things enough for the check to tear out cleanly.

Checks & Credit cards

You may already have had difficulty signing credit card slips and checks. If so, please turn to page *176, for help* **Signing your name**.

Spring-loaded Faucets

It's aggravating the first time you single-handedly face a ***Spring-Loaded, Auto-Shutoff Faucet*** in a public restroom. In case you haven't met one yet, it's a single warm water faucet for each washbasin. Sounds good so far, doesn't it? One hand, one faucet...

The problem with these is that the handle is spring-loaded which allows water to flow only when your one hand twists or presses the handle. As soon as you release the handle to slide your one hand under the running water, the water shuts off!

It doesn't work to plug the drain with paper towels so you can fill the bowl with water. It just makes a mess. But you can turn the faucet on high, so the volume of water gushing into the bowl exceeds that draining out.

Half-fill the sink bowl and dip your one hand into the water. Soap, and rinse while the water drains out. To make this work, you do have to wash rather quickly.

You may never run into these. Recent trends in restroom plumbing are tending toward *Timed-Flow* and *-Sensor* faucets These turn on and off, often with minimal input from you.

Serving board

I remember watching my one-handed grandfather, Duke (*see page 5*), serve cocktails to his guests at family gatherings. To do it, he used a wooden serving tray shaped like a paddle which he'd customized with two rows of three beveled indents perfectly fitted to his cocktail glasses. He took drink orders in the other rooms, mixed the drinks in the kitchen, arranged the glasses on the tray, and then circulated among his guests telling people, "*Jack, yours is the left column, center row.*" While he walked around serving drinks, he carried his own drink tucked into his shirt pocket.

Umbrellas

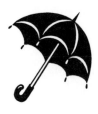

An automatic push button umbrella is the obvious solution to single-handling an umbrella while staying dry. Of course, automatic umbrellas heavier to carry and a bit more expensive.

You can also manage a regular manual umbrella with one hand.

Leaving the umbrella strap fastened, pick up your umbrella by the handle, as if to shake hands with it, holding as close to the end of the handle as possible and with the tip pointing skyward. Firmly flick your wrist downward, extending the umbrella shaft to its full length. (*Alternatively, hold the umbrella by the handle and bring the cloth end up under your armpit. Pinch it there. Straighten your elbow to extend the umbrella shaft.)*

Now slide your one hand down the shaft, about halfway, swinging the umbrella baton-like. With the handle now trapped under the armpit of the hand you use unfasten the strap. Slide the metal collar center of the ribs, toward the tip of the shaft, stretching out the umbrella until the ring clicks through its hook, locking the umbrella open.

After the rain, to close your umbrella rest the handle against your sternum (*your "breastbone"*). Sliding your hand along the shaft while also supporting the umbrella, reach inside the open umbrella and unclasp the hook that locks the collar in place. Now slide the collar down the shaft, closing the umbrella.

If, when using your umbrella on a windy day, the wind blows your umbrella in-side-out, you can fix this problem easily, by pointing the tip of the umbrella into the wind. This way, the wind blows your umbrella right-side-out.

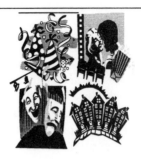

LEISURE ACTIVITIES

Many more activities are still open to single-handed-you than you may have thought. The adaptations and theory already described in this book also apply to what you do on your own time—for fun. With some planning, you can probably continue participating in whatever activities you've always enjoyed.

Cards

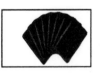

Even convicted criminals on Death Row play cards—so there's no reason why you shouldn't enjoy them too, even single-handedly.

We were a cribbage family. After a spring vacation week with Dad's parents, I came home nearly convinced *"fifteen-two, fifteen-four, fifteen-six, a pair for eight, a run for eleven, and the jack of nobs for twelve"* was the only way to count.

The two issues to playing cards with one hand are *Shuffling*, and *Holding your cards* for study and when you play them.

Holding cards.

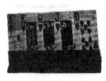

Card Racks, look like a larger version of a *Scrabble* letter rack and free your one hand for play-making. A card rack allows you to arrange a hand of cards on the table in front of you but also to keep your hand out of your opponent's sight. Wooden or plastic, a card rack is a shelf with a beveled ridge slot to fit the card bottom edges into. Your cards then lean against the back of the rack without sliding out

Shuffling cards

When playing a two-handed opponent, s/he *could* take care of all the shuffling This is your "quick & dirty" *no-cost* solution.

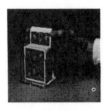

A **Card Shuffler** (*pictured left*) is an open top plastic box somewhat deeper than a deck of cards, with a stable base enabling it to stand upright while in use.

To use your card shuffler, fill the box with two-thirds of the deck. Then push the remaining third of the deck into the shuffler amongst the two thirds of the deck already in the holder. Remove a different third of the cards and repeat the process four or five times.

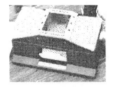

Battery operated *automatic card shufflers* shuffle up to two decks of cards at the push of a button. It works by rotating like a Ferris wheel, depositing cards, shuffling

them on the *seats* with each turn. If your one hand isn't your dominant hand, this may be your solution.

Hand Crafts

Using adaptive equipment as necessary, even single-handedly you can continue enjoying many hand crafts usually considered two-handed projects.

Embroidery

If you happily embroidered two-handedly, there's no reason not to continue. And if you've never embroidered, want to try?

Place the bottom half of your embroidery hoop on the table (*Metal embroidery hoops clamp over the cloth more easily, and hold more tightly than do lighter weight wooden ones.*) and lay the material over that bottom half of your embroidery hoop. Clamp the top half of the hoop over the material, pressing it firmly over the material and onto the bottom half of the embroidery hoop.

With the material snugly trapped inside the embroidery hoop, hold the hoop horizontal, with the stenciled embroidery pattern facing the hand you use, by catching just enough of the hoop rim, between your knees, to hold it steady. Just press your knees together to hold the hoop. You will be working on your embroidery sideways, but can make the position a bit more comfortable for yourself by adjusting your upper body.

* * * * *

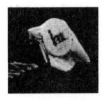

You can also try using an adapted embroidery hoop, (*pictured left*) which is fitted with an adjustable stand that clamps to the arm of your chair or to the edge of a table, enabling you to work on your embroidery straight on, as if you had an *other* hand *holding the hoop.*

Knitting and Crocheting

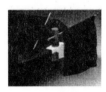

Two-handed knitters and *crocheters* use both hands, manipulating the crochet hook with one and the yarn with another, or by moving one knitting needle with one hand and the yarn and second needle with the other. Single-handedly, use a *knitting needle/crochet hook holder* clamped to the chair arm or to a table. You knit by manipulating the yarn and the other needle around the stabilized knitting needle, or crochet by manipulating yarn around the stabilized crochet hook.

Reading

Reading is another of the activities that even criminals can pursue, so why not you? Losing use of one hand mustn't keep you from enjoying a book, magazine, or newspaper whenever you want.

Books

For many years probably, you've enjoyed reading. Quite naturally, you'd like to be able to read where ever you are, *even while one-handed.* Maybe you've always read while waiting in line, while commuting to work, or simply traveling—on subways, trains, and planes. Or maybe you enjoy curling up on the couch with a good book... You want to be able to read whether you're standing, sitting, or even while eating, even while your one handed.

If you've already tried reading single-handedly, you've run into **The Problem:** *You must always hold the book open with your one hand.* Every time you move that one hand, to do anything else, the already read pages flip back over to the other side, onto the ones you've not yet read.

It doesn't matter whether you move your hand to adjust your glasses, take a bite of sandwich, rub your eyes, raise your coffee to your lips, or to mark a phrase with your highlighter... There are ways to deal with this.

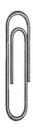

Paperclip For public transportation reading, and other *out-of-home* reading, clip a jumbo Paperclip to the top of the last four or five pages you've read. The weight of the Paperclip will keep the pages from flipping closed when you *need* to move your one hand. You can also use a 1¾" Butterfly -Paperclips. Butterfly Paperclips are heavier and clip more pages, so they're even more effective.

Bookminder Try this clever tool (*pictured left*) for at-home reading The *Bookminder* holds your book open by holding pages under its clear plastic flexible flaps. With this design, you can read even the words under the plastic flaps. *For information on obtaining a Bookminder see* **Resources**, *page 246.*

Hands-Free Reading is another gadget designed to hold your book open. It looks like a metal comb but with four, three inch prongs.

Hands-Free Reading is a bit more difficult to set up than the *Bookminder*. With the book open, slide the outside prongs under the first and the last pages of the book—the inside prongs rest on the left and right open pages. Turning each page, and re-setting up, after reading the two open pages is an interruption, but after a while you may become adept. ***Hands-Free Reading*** *is rather a catch-as-catch-can item. Here and there bookstores stock this item at the register counter.*

Newspapers

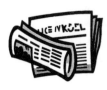

Two-handed people read newspapers fully opened out and held between their *two* hands.

Not only are newspaper pages over-sized, but they're loose, and laid-out with articles continuing from page one, onto page twelve, or deeper, and not always even the same section... Single-handed newspaper reading calls for creativity, and some *body positioning*.

To successfully read your newspaper single-handedly, sit down at a table or desk. You need to be able to spread the paper out open flat, in front of you. Those cute little tables in cafes and coffee shops are almost big enough but only if you move the sugar, salt, and pepper shakers, the *specials* tent card, and the rest of the stuff set out for your convenience, onto one of the *extra* chairs beside you. If you also want to sip a cup of coffee while you read, you'll need to keep another *extra* chair close so you don't have to keep lifting your cup off the open newspaper whenever you turn the page.

* * * * *

Alternatively, New York commuters have a method for reading the New York Times or Wall Street Journal, even inside crowded trains. They do it by *setting up* each section and reading the paper one section at a time. *Set-up* a section by unfolding the center fold so the whole front page opens in front of you. Then fold the section in half, lengthwise making a long narrow three-column strip of newspaper to contend with. You read the paper in three column swatches, and don't turn to inside pages to continue a story.

The commuter train method works single-handedly, if you rest your paper against a table while you read. The advantage is that it allows you to still fit your coffee cup on the table while you read, or to share the table with someone else, even if it's a smallish table.

Pool

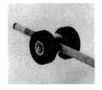

No, shooting pool isn't only for the bi-handed. You *can* shoot single-handedly, *with the assistance of a piece of equipment.* Obviously, you'll need help supporting the cue while you line up and make your shots single-handedly. For that, all you need is a Cue Bridge (*pictured, left*). With practice, you can learn to setup your cue bridge for any shot.

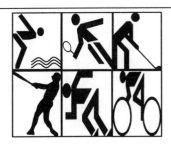

SPORTS

Perhaps you awoke in a hospital room, like I did, to contemplate living the rest of your life single-handedly. Maybe you believed you had to write off actually being involved athletically, and imagined your sporting future as nothing more than long sedentary days just *spectating*.

Or you may be looking at recuperation from a temporary loss of the use of one hand, and be wondering if you'll have to forgo all of it, except for watching sports happen around you.

Not so.

Since my hemorrhage, more than nineteen years ago, I've skied *black diamond* trails, played some mean ping pong, run a 10K and a marathon, golfed. (*I'm not a golfer, but I did try*.) I've seen some fast single-handed tennis, and competitive sailing. Not only are sports great exercise—critical to *good health*—but sports are an excellent way to meet people. You don't need to be the best at it, "*a super-gimp,*" you only have to be good enough to get out there and have fun trying.

Disabled Sports USA

If you've permanently lost the use of your *other* hand, as a person with disability, you can take advantage of unique opportunities to relearn a sport or to learn new recreational and competitive sporting activity, by networking socially and meeting others with disability, people who are already participating in activities despite a wide variety of disability and disabling conditions.

If you are an individual with long-term disability, you are eligible to become a member of *Disabled Sports USA. DS/USA* is a nonprofit organization with regional affiliate branches dedicated to teaching, organizing, and promoting handicapped sports all around the country.

This all-volunteer web of associations is devoted to improving and increasing sporting and recreational opportunities for people with disability. The national office, located outside Washington DC, can direct you to a local group of people with disabled and able-bodied volunteers near you who have experience in adapting equipment as necessary to get you participating in the sports and activities you've decided to try.

Disabled Sports USA will be able to put you in touch with the local group that can help you learn how to participate in the activities that interest you. To hook up with the DS/USA affiliate nearest you, contact Disabled Sports USA by calling, writing, or logging on:

Disabled Sports/USA
451 Hungerford Drive, Suite. 100
Rockville, MD 20850
301/217-0960
http://www.dsusa.org

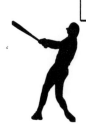

Baseball

If Jim Abbott, who has started with the California Angels and New York Yankees, can pitch major league baseball with one hand, you can play too. Watch how he does it—If it's off-season, check out a game video. He perches his glove on his stump while throwing. As he releases the ball, he slides his one hand back into his *perched* mitt, so he's ready to field a bunt or a line drive back. Since childhood, Jim Abbott used creativity and ingenuity to enable him to play the game he loves.

If you don't have a stump on which you could reliably hang your mitt, what if you made a sort of belt, or attached a perch to your trousers? If you really want to play, you *can* do it single-handedly.

Bowling

Even post-stroke, despite diminished function in one leg, _if that's a problem_, you can enjoy candlestick bowling. You can also pick up the larger and heavier Tenpin balls from the rack. Place the four fingers and thumb of your one hand into the finger holes in the ball. Then rest the ball on your hip while you walk into position. Of course, The smaller candlepin balls will be easier to manage single-handedly.

Bowling is inherently a one-handed sport with the _other_ hand (_if you had the use of another one_) only minimally involved, to help with picking up or carrying the ball.

However, bowling won't feel the same as it did before you lost the use of your hand/arm. Because your upper body is integral to maintaining and monitoring balance, you'll probably feel awkward, almost as though you've forgotten something, the first few times you pick up the ball to take your place behind the line, and make those few forceful run/walk steps.

Well, you have "_forgotten_" something. You've "_forgotten_" to use your _other_ hand. That's okay. Bowling is still infinitely doable. You'll get used to the balance-thing.

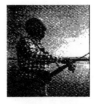

Fishing

You thought you'd be facing an angling-free life? Would I do that to you? Of course not! An ***Angler's Aid Rod Holster*** (*pictured left*) enables you to single-handedly fight the fish you've hooked. It's been "field-tested" and truly makes single-handed fishing infinitely doable.

You'll continue to cast single handedly, but now you can fight the fish and reel it in yourself, too. With the butt of your rod held in the holster, your one hand is free to reel in your catch.

Golf

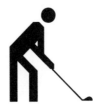

All golfers spend hours developing the swings that land the ball where it has to go to play the course. If you learned a comfortable two-handed stroke, you can develop a one-handed stroke. Don't forget the first two *Secrets, on page 11, Body Positioning* and *Four Fingers & a Thumb.*

Try using your whole arm to hold and steady the golf club. Try gripping your club with a hold similar to the one described for handling a broom and sweeping, (*see page 167*). Maybe you'll need to try different club weights and lengths. Chances are the golf pro at your club will be intrigued by the thought of adapting the game for single-handed play, and interested in helping you develop solutions that enable you to improve your game. Don't hesitate to ask. Those deeply involved in a sport or hobby often welcome challenges testing their expertise.

Running

You're probably thinking, *"of course I can still run. I damaged my arm (my hand) not my foot!"* And yes, you probably still can run. However, consider these few things.

Balance: First, as upright creatures, our arms and hands are integral elements in maintaining our balance. Swinging our arms when we move is part of that balance maintenance, but more to the point, over the years, each of us has grown accustomed to our own unique carriage, and that carriage is the basis for our individual sense of balance. After losing the use of a hand or arm, your body needs to *"recalibrate"* your sense of balance. Before you go out running, do check to see that *"recalibration"* is well enough along.

Shoes: Secondly, most running shoes lace-up. In order to put on your shoes, you'll need to prepare them for one-handed tying by relacing them (*see page 72*). Because securely tied shoes are important for running, you'll want to practice tying your shoes and put off running until you're adept at the one-handed shoe tie.

Reflectors: Third, if you plan to run in the evening and your reflector vest ties at the hip and under your arms, unless you can leave it tied, and slip it on overhead, you're going to want another vest. Look for one with Velcro, snap, hook, or buckle fasteners.

Sweatband: Slip on your headband single-handedly by holding the band in the back and catching the front on your forehead, by trapping the headband against a door jamb or utility pole. And adjust the back making the headband comfortable.

Skiing

In that skiing is mainly a "leg" sport, you probably expect that you can continue skiing after losing the use of your arm and or hand, and you're probably right. As with most sports, skiing is highly dependent on good balance, and as discussed above in **Running/*Balance*,** losing the use of your hand or arm affects your balance (*See above for a longer discussion.*)

The main difference between skiing single-handedly and with two hands, is that you'll only have one pole.

Many skiers learned to "*unweight*" by planting the left ski pole to turn left, and the right pole to turn right. If with two hands you were taught, and continued to use your ski poles when initiating and completing your turns, this will be the most difficult part about re-learning to ski single-handedly. You *can* re-learn, but while you're learning, undoubtedly you'll leave a lot of "*sitzmarks*" on the slopes, scatter a few "*yard sales*" behind you, and generate some mighty "*blizzards*" while your at it. Be prepared.

Swimming

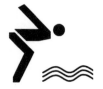

Swimming is wonderful muscle toning exercise. Your buoyancy in water can also be good therapy if there's possibility that with effort you might regain the use of that *other* hand or arm.

You'll notice that single-handedly your swimming feels uneven. Of course! Even if you *can* use your shoulder and arm, if you can't cup the water with your *other* hand, and you do with your one hand, you'll be uneven. Experiment with different strokes, the "lifesaving" side-stroke works single-handedly, since the lifesaver is supposed to reserve the *other* hand to bring in the "life being saved." If you're one-armed *and* one-handed, this might be the perfect stroke for you.

Table Tennis

There's plenty of room between your palm and paddle handle to hold a ping pong ball. Drop the ball to the table. Hit it off the first bounce and you've served. After service, ping pong is a one-handed sport, even if you have two hands.

Tennis

Serving is the real two-handed crux of tennis. Try serving by holding the ball in the palm of your one hand, pressed against the racket handle, and practice tossing it up from that hand-hold and hitting it. Single-handedly, you may not play a professional circuit. But then again...

Volleyball

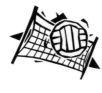

Volleyball is infinitely Single-*handleable.* Serve by palming the ball and pushing it up into the air. Hit it over the net on its way back down, directing it to the hole in the defense by pressing with one or more of your fingers or thumb (*the Second Secret, remember? see page 12*).

Keep in mind that *Second Secret. (You don't have "only" one-hand. You have four fingers and a thumb.)* If you always make use of those four fingers and thumb every time the ball is yours to hit, and if you position your body so your four fingers and thumb are always lined up to whack that ball to where the other team isn't expecting it, you'll be one of the first players selected to a team.

SEXUALITY

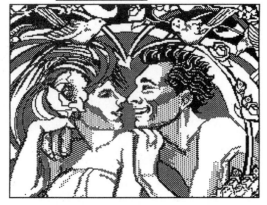

As far as I'm concerned one-handedness is irrelevant to sexuality. Great sex should be a *whole you* experience—a body-mind-spirit exploration.

The fact of the matter is: It's what you do with what do you have, how you use what you have that makes great sex, not what you don't have or don't do.

It isn't appropriate for me to map out the mechanics of sex here. This isn't meant to be a sex manual. Many others, with longer pedigrees in the discipline than I, address step-by-step discussions of satisfying yourself and your partner.

My primary purpose is to assure you that your single-handed sex life can not only be satisfactory, but even exemplary. Sexuality isn't a two-handed thing.

The dexterity of that hand you use, improved by demands single-handedness places on it, coupled with your experience in substituting body positioning for an *other hand* can make a satisfying sex life, with or without a partner, very much available to you.

In this era of Sexually Transmitted Diseases (STDs) and particularly HIV/ AIDS, I feel it would be irresponsible to open up a discussion of sexuality without mentioning safe sex, and in particular, condoms.

Single-handedly, why not integrate condoms into foreplay? Why not make safe sex part of your sexual experience, an integral part of foreplay and intimacy?

Heterosexually speaking, if your partner holds the foil condom package, you can tear it open. If your partner picks out the condom, laying it over the penis, you can roll it down, or vise versa. Sharing the responsibility, and taking it together, makes using a condom a part of and climactic to foreplay.

Whatever your sexual preference, make protecting yourself a seamless part of your sensual experience.

Most importantly, enjoying your sexuality single-handedly means, rather than focusing on *"just one hand,"* focusing on the *Second Secret*, four fingers and a thumb. Each one of those four fingers and thumb. With all your practice, you easily accomplish more with those four fingers which are stronger and more dexterous, than are the fingers of two hands.

My final advise regarding single-handed sexuality is simply this; *"Relax."* If you take the time to select and to get to know your partner, you'll probably find *you're* more hung-up about your one-handedness than your partner is.

Think about it for a second. If your one-handedness was a problem for your partner, s/he probably wouldn't be there with you in the first place. If you want to be active sexually, your single-handedness should not be the barrier. Finding someone worth the experience should be the only barrier to your sexuality

But please. *Please*. ***Please***. Things are hard enough when you're managing single-handedly—***Please*** practice safe sex.

EPILOGUE

As you go about life with your new attitude toward *"two-handed operations"* and your new approach to managing single-handedly, I have no doubt that you'll develop your own solutions to obstacles I didn't touch on here. Every day, I'm trying something different. Managing single-handedly is a learning, growing process.

I'm always open to new ideas, and I love sharing in the successes of my comrades in single-handedness. I welcome the opportunity to hear from you. Tell me about conundrums you face down, and about how you overcame the *insurmountable*. Please write to me about your successes, care of my publisher:

> Prince Gallison Press
> PO Box 23, Hanover Station
> Boston, MA 02113-0001
> E-mail: ***princeg@gis.net***
> ***http://www.gis.net/princeg***

I truly do look forward to hearing from you. And I hope you found my book helped you to get back into the business of participating in your life again.

Tom

RESOURCES

Pg. #	Product	Company & Product Number
236	Angler's Aid Rod Holster	Access to Recreation, #RH101
230	Bookminder	Titan Pro, Inc.
129	Box Top Opener	Alimed, Inc. #8611
16	Buff Puff Back Scrub **Shower Brush**	Available in most **health and beauty stores** or store sections.
52	Button Hook (Aid)	TheraPro, Inc., #DLD0603 Sammons Preston, #BK 2008 North Coast Medical #NC28667 Alimed, #8258
131	Can Opener	Sammons-Preston, #E3047 North Coast Medical #NC28220
226	Card Rack,	Sammons Preston, #9434 North Coast Medical # NC29106 Alimed, Inc. #8300
226	Card Shuffler (Automatic)	Sammons-Preston, #E9424
110	Cut-up Knife	Sammons-Preston #BK1410
232	Cue Bridge	Access to Recreation, #ML63
120	Cutting Board	TheraPro, Inc., #DLK0602 Sammons-Preston #3044 North Coast Med. #NC28503 Alimed, Inc.#8178
44	Dressing Stick	TheraPro, Inc., #DLD0601 Sammons-Preston #E2109 North Coast Medical #NC28575 Alimed, Inc.#8269
129	Dycem	TheraPro (various product numbers) Sammons-Preston (var. product #'s) North Coast Medical(var. product #s) Alimed, Inc. (various product numbers)

Page#	Product	Company & Product Number
227	Embroidery/ Crochet Holder	North Coast Medical, #NC28862
39	Flossers	*Available where ever dental supplies are sold*
127	Food Processor	*Available where ever kitchen and cooking appliances are sold.*
15	Grab Bar	TheraPro, various models. Alimed, Inc. various models
124	Grater	*Available where cooking supplies are sold.*
29	Hair Dryer Holder	Sammons Preston #6483
190	Half-QWERTY	The Matias Corporation.
131	Hand-held Can Opener	Sammons-Preston, Inc. #3047 North Coast Medical #NC8220
127	Hand held mixer	Black & Decker: *Available where ever cooking appliances are sold.*
16	Handled Bath Sponge	TheraPro, Inc., #LB0901 North Coast Medical, #NC28645 Alimed, Inc. #8536
133	Jar/Lid opener, #NC28214	Sammons-Preston # E3088 North Coast Medical, #NC28214 Alimed, Inc. #8268
140	Kitchen Soap Dispenser	*Available where ever kitchen and plumbing supplies are sold*
228	Knitting needle Holder	Sammons-Preston, Inc.
45	L'eggs Pantyhose	OneHanesPlace
30	Nail Care Center.	Sammons-Preston. #E6298-03
125	Pan holder	Sammons-Preston, #E3011 North Coast Medical #NC28221 Alimed, Inc. #8280

Pg. #	Product	Company & Product Number
191	Personal Keyboard	Infogrip, Inc.
109	Rocker Knife	TheraPro, Inc., #DLE0612 Sammons Preston, #BK1405 North Coast Med., #NC229272 Alimed, Inc. #8116
126	Roller Knife	Sammons-Preston, #1399 North Coast Medical #NC65601
95	Spreading Board	North Coast Medical #NC35789
191	Step On It, computer foot pedals	Bilbo Innovations Inc.
206	Steering Wheel Knob	North Coast Medical #NC90100
126	Suction cup pad *"Little Octopus"*	Sammons-Preston, #1259 Alimed, Inc. #8265
199	Telephone Headset	*Available at telephony or office supplies stores*
38	Toothpaste dispenser System Page	Sammons-Preston, Inc. #E3348
190	*Type With One Hand, by Nina Richardson 82752*	Access to Recreation, #BK96 South-Western Ed. Publishing
26	Velcro Curlers	Wilhold and Goody, *Available in most health and beauty stores and sections of chain drug stores*
71	Velcro Shoes	Wissota Traders
196	Voice Recognition computer equipment	*Your best bet is to check out your local computer superstore.* *Or search the Web.*
90	Winged Cork Screw	*Available in most kitchen and cooking stores and sections of chain housewares stores*

SUPPLIERS OF GADGETS DISCUSSED:

- **Access to Recreation,** 2509 Thousand Oaks Blvd., Suite 430, Thousand Oaks, CA 91362 1-800-634-4351, http://www.quadcontrol.com

- **Bilbo Innovations Inc.**, 1290 Oakmead Pkwy, #118, Sunnyvale, CA 94086, 1-408-736-6086, http://www.bilbo.com/bilbo.html

- **Infogrip, Inc.**, 1141 East Main St., Ventura, CA 93001, 1-800-397-0921, http://www.infogrip.com

- **The Matias Corporation,** 100 Rexdale Blvd., Suite 1204, Rexdale, ON CANADA M9W 6T4, 1-888-ONE-HAND http://www.dgp.toronto.edu/matias/product.html

- **North Coast Med.,** P.O. Box 6070,San Jose, CA 95150, http://www.ncMed.com

- **OneHanesPlace,** P.O. Box 00748, Rural Hall, NC 27098, 1-800-300-2600, http://www.ohpcatalog.com

- **Prince Gallison Press,** P.O. Box 23—Hanover Station, Boston, MA 02113-0001 1-617-367-5815 http://www.gis.net/princeg

- **Sammons-Preston,** P.O. Box 32, Brookfield, IL 60513, 1-800-323-5547 http://www.sammonspreston.com

[continued...]

- **South-Western Educational Publishing,**
  5101 Madison Rd., Cincinnati, OH 45227
  1-513-527-9221 http://www.swep.com

- **Therapro, Inc.**, 225 Arlington St., Framingham, MA
  01702-8723, 1-800-2570-5376
  http://www.theraproducts.com

- **Titan Pro, Inc.**, 1430 Koll Circle, Suite 108, San
  Jose, CA 95112, 408-437-5471
  http://www.i-netmall.com/shops/titan/

- **Wissota Traders,** 1313 1st Avenue, Chippewa Falls,
  WI 54729-149, 1-800-833-6421, No WEBsite found.

ABOUT THE AUTHOR

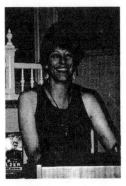

Also by Tommye-K. Mayer,"*Teaching Me To Run* © *2001,* Prince Gallison Press. is Mayer's memoir about how and why she taught her stroke paralyzed body to run. The story culminates with finishing Boston's Tufts 10K.

Tommye-Karen Mayer is an experienced speaker. Mayer may be available to address your organization's next conference. To make arrangements contact Prince Gallison Press at:

P.O. Box 23, Hanover Station
Boston, MA 02113-0001
 princeg@gis.net
617-367-5815 (tel)
617-367-3337

Mayer has a BA in Sociology from Wheaton College, Norton Massachusetts. The year after graduation she began graduate work in Rehabilitation through the "School of Hard Knocks" when she survived a nearly fatal thalamic cerebral hemorrhage. Mayer has been working on rehabilitating herself ever since; Especially after a negligent automobile driver drove over her affected left foot returning her to complete left hemi-paresis ten years after the hemorrhage/stroke.